Preventive Medicine

Editor

STEPHANIE L. NEARY

PHYSICIAN ASSISTANT CLINICS

www.physicianassistant.theclinics.com

Consulting Editor
JAMES A. VAN RHEE

January 2022 • Volume 7 • Number 1

ELSEVIER

1600 John F. Kennedy Boulevard • Suite 1800 • Philadelphia, Pennsylvania, 19103-2899

http://www.theclinics.com

PHYSICIAN ASSISTANT CLINICS Volume 7, Number 1
January 2022 ISSN 2405-7991, ISBN-13: 978-0-323-83534-3

Editor: Katerina Heidhausen
Developmental Editor: Axell Ivan Jade Purificacion

Physician Assistant Clinics (ISSN: 2405–7991) is published quarterly by Elsevier Inc., 360 Park Avenue South, New York, NY 10010-1710. Months of issue are January, April, July, and October. Periodicals postage paid at New York, NY and additional mailing offices. Subscription prices are $150.00 per year (US individuals), $305.00 (US institutions), $100.00 (US students), $150.00 (Canadian individuals), $320.00 (Canadian institutions), $100.00 (Canadian students), $150.00 (international individuals), $320.00 (international institutions), and $100.00 (international students). Foreign air speed delivery is included in all *Clinics* subscription prices. All prices are subject to change without notice. POSTMASTER: Send address changes to *Physician Assistant Clinics*, Elsevier Periodicals Customer Service, 11830 Westline Industrial Drive, St. Louis, MO 63146. Customer Service Health Sciences Division, Subscription Customer Service, 3251 Riverport Lane, Maryland Heights, MO 63043. **Customer Service: 1-800-654-2452 (U.S. and Canada); 314-447-8871 (outside U.S. and Canada). Fax: 314-447-8029. E-mail: journalscustomerservice-usa@elsevier.com (for print support); journalsonlinesupport-usa@elsevier.com (for online support).**

Reprints. For copies of 100 or more, of articles in this publication, please contact the Commercial Reprints Department, Elsevier Inc., 360 Park Avenue South, New York, NY 10010-1710. Tel. 212-633-3874; Fax: 212-633-3820; E-mail: reprints@elsevier.com.

Physician Assistant Clinics is covered in *EMBASE/Excerpta Medica* and *ESCI*.

PROGRAM OBJECTIVE
The goal of the Physician Assistant Clinics is to keep practicing physician assistants up to date with current clinical practice by providing timely articles reviewing the state of the art in patient care.

TARGET AUDIENCE
Physician Assistants and other healthcare professionals

LEARNING OBJECTIVES
Upon completion of this activity, participants will be able to:
1. Review common preventative health topics and actions.
2. Discuss advocating for change in communities and healthcare systems.
3. Recognize how policy change impacts healthcare.

ACCREDITATION
The Elsevier Office of Continuing Medical Education (EOCME) is accredited by the Accreditation Council for Continuing Medical Education (ACCME) to provide continuing medical education for physicians.

The EOCME designates this journal-based CME activity for a maximum of 15 *AMA PRA Category 1 Credit*(s)™. Physicians should claim only the credit commensurate with the extent of their participation in the activity.

All other healthcare professionals requesting continuing education credit for this enduring material will be issued a certificate of participation.

DISCLOSURE OF CONFLICTS OF INTEREST
The EOCME assesses conflict of interest with its instructors, faculty, planners, and other individuals who are in a position to control the content of CME activities. All relevant conflicts of interest that are identified are thoroughly vetted by EOCME for fair balance, scientific objectivity, and patient care recommendations. EOCME is committed to providing its learners with CME activities that promote improvements or quality in healthcare and not a specific proprietary business or a commercial interest.

The planning committee, staff, authors, and editors listed below have identified no financial relationships or relationships to products or devices they or their spouse/life partner have with commercial interest related to the content of this CME activity:
Megan S. Ady, MSPAS, PA-C; Esther Bennitta; Kari S. Bernard, PA-C, PhD; Scott Carlson, DO, MPH; Andrew P. Chastain, MSPAS, PA-C; Regina Chavous-Gibson, MSN, RN; DeShana Collett, PA-C, PhD; Emily B. Douglas, MSPAS, PA-C; David T. Dubé, DHSc, MSc, PA-C; Kenneth Early, CPNP-AC; Nicole Ferschke, MMS, MBS, PA-C; Gina L. Hogg, MSPAS, PA-C, GMPA, SCAPA, AAPA; Eve B. Hoover, DMSc, MS, PA-C, DFAAPA; Aislinn E. Hopkins, MSPAS, PA-C; Stephanie Jalaba, MMS, PA-C; Pollyanna Kabara, EdD, MS, PA-C; Sarah Dion Kelly, MMSc, PA-C, RDN, CDCES; Jonathan Kilstrom, MPAS, PA-C, NRP; Aimee Lamb, PA-C, MMSs; Melanie M. Lyon, MSPAS, PA-C; Joel G. McReynolds, PA-C, MPAS, CAQ-Orthopedic Surgery; Stephanie L. Neary, MPA, MMS, PA-C; Nguyen H. Park, MS, PA-C, DFAAPA; Sarah Pieper, MPAS, PA-C; Charles Regan, MS, PA-C; Lauren Richardson, MSM, PA-C; Matéa M. Rippe, MPAS, PA-C; Tia M. Solh, MT(ASCP), MSPAS, PA-C; Kay Miller Temple, MD, MMC; Heather Trudeau, MPAS, PA-C; James A. Van Rhee, MS, PA-C; Roger D. Wells, PA-C; Anne Wildermuth, MMS, PA-C, EM CAQ, RD; Matthew Wright, MS, PA-C, RD; Jennifer Simms Zorn, DMS, PA-C

UNAPPROVED/OFF-LABEL USE DISCLOSURE
The EOCME requires CME faculty to disclose to the participants:
1. When products or procedures being discussed are off-label, unlabelled, experimental, and/or investigational (not US Food and Drug Administration [FDA] approved); and
2. Any limitations on the information presented, such as data that are preliminary or that represent ongoing research, interim analyses, and/or unsupported opinions. Faculty may discuss information about pharmaceutical agents that is outside of FDA-approved labelling. This information is intended solely for CME and is not intended to promote off-label use of these medications. If you have any questions, contact the medical affairs department of the manufacturer for the most recent prescribing information.

TO ENROLL
The CME program is available to all Physician Assistant Clinics subscribers at no additional fee. To subscribe to the Physician Assistant Clinics, call customer service at 1-800-654-2452 or sign up online at www.physicianassistant.theclinics.com.

METHOD OF PARTICIPATION

In order to claim credit, participants must complete the following:

1. Complete enrolment as indicated above
2. Read the activity
3. Complete the CME Test and Evaluation. Participants must achieve a score of 70% on the test. All CME Tests and Evaluations must be completed online

CME INQUIRIES/SPECIAL NEEDS

For all CME inquiries or special needs, please contact elsevierCME@elsevier.com.

Contributors

CONSULTING EDITOR

JAMES A. VAN RHEE, MS, PA-C
Associate Professor, Program Director, Yale School of Medicine, Yale Physician Assistant Online Program, New Haven, Connecticut

EDITOR

STEPHANIE L. NEARY, MPA, MMS, PA-C
Assistant Professor Adjunct, Director of Didactic Education, Yale Physician Assistant Online Program, New Haven, Connecticut

AUTHORS

MEGAN S. ADY, MSPAS, PA-C
Assistant Professor, Division of Physician Assistant Studies, Murphy Deming College of Health Sciences at Mary Baldwin University, Fishersville, Virginia

KARI S. BERNARD, PA-C, PhD
Associate Director of Research and Capstone Activities, A.T. Still University, Arizona School of Health Sciences, Associate Professor, Doctor of Medical Science Program, Psychiatric PA, Orion Behavioral Health Network, Anchorage, Alaska

SCOTT CARLSON, DO, MPH
Medical Director, Department of PA Medicine, Michigan State University College of Osteopathic Medicine, East Lansing, Michigan

ANDREW P. CHASTAIN, MSPAS, PA-C
Assistant Professor, Medical Science and Physician Assistant Studies Department, Butler University, Indianapolis, Indiana

DESHANA COLLETT, PA-C, PhD
Professor, Department of Physician Assistant Studies, University of Kentucky College of Health Sciences, Lexington, Kentucky

EMILY B. DOUGLAS, MSPAS, PA-C
Instructor in the Division of Physician Assistant Studies, College of Health Professions, Medical University of South Carolina, Charleston, South Carolina

DAVID T. DUBÉ, DHSc, MSc, PA-C
Assistant Clinical Professor, Physician Assistant Program, University of New England, Portland, Maine

KENNETH EARLY, CPNP-AC
Assistant Professor, LTU Physician Assistant Program, Department of Natural Sciences, College of Arts and Sciences, Lawrence Technological University, Southfield, Michigan

NICOLE FERSCHKE, MMS, MBS, PA-C
Clinical Assistant Professor, Clinical Coordinator, Department of Physician Assistant Studies, Northern Arizona University, Phoenix Biomedical Campus, Phoenix, Arizona

GINA L. HOGG, MSPAS, PA-C, GMPA, SCAPA, AAPA
Geriatric Medicine Physician Assistant, Internal Medicine and Geriatrics, Medical University of South Carolina, Charleston, South Carolina

EVE B. HOOVER, DMSc, MS, PA-C, DFAAPA
Associate Professor, Midwestern University PA Program, Glendale, Arizona

AISLINN E. HOPKINS, MSPAS, PA-C
Instructor in the Division of Physician Assistant Studies, College of Health Professions, Medical University of South Carolina, Charleston, South Carolina

STEPHANIE JALABA, MMS, PA-C
Assistant Professor, Department of PA Medicine, Michigan State University College of Osteopathic Medicine, East Lansing, Michigan

POLLYANNA KABARA, EdD, MS, PA-C
Lakeside Pediatrics, Children's Wisconsin, Milwaukee, Wisconsin

SARAH DION KELLY, MMSc, PA-C, RDN, CDCES
Inova Cares Clinic for Families, Sterling, Virginia

JONATHAN KILSTROM, MPAS, PA-C, NRP
Instructor, Yale College of Medicine, Physician Assistant Online Program, New Haven, Connecticut

AIMEE LAMB, PA-C, MMSs
Program Director, LTU Physician Assistant Program, Department of Natural Sciences, College of Arts and Sciences, Lawrence Technological University, Southfield, Michigan

MELANIE M. LYON, MSPAS, PA-C
Physician Assistant, Neighborhood Outreach Access to Health – HonorHealth, Phoenix, Arizona

JOEL G. MCREYNOLDS, PA-C, MPAS, CAQ-Orthopedic Surgery
New West Sports Medicine and Orthopedic Surgery, Kearney, Nebraska

NGUYEN H. PARK, MS, PA-C, DFAAPA
President/Founder, Society of Physician Assistants in Genetics/Genomics, Great Falls, Virginia

SARAH PIEPER, MPAS, PA-C
Concordia University Wisconsin, Mequon, Wisconsin

CHARLES REGAN, MS, PA-C
Assistant Professor, LTU Physician Assistant Program, Department of Natural Sciences, College of Arts and Sciences, Lawrence Technological University, Southfield, Michigan

LAUREN RICHARDSON, MSM, PA-C
South College, School of Physician Assistant Studies, Principal Faculty, Knoxville, Tennessee

MATÉA M. RIPPE, MPAS, PA-C
Indianapolis, Indiana

TIA M. SOLH, MT(ASCP), MSPAS, PA-C
Department of Physician Assistant Studies, South College - Atlanta Campus, Atlanta, Georgia

KAY MILLER TEMPLE, MD, MMC
Rural Health Information Hub, Center for Rural Health, University of North Dakota School of Medicine and Health Sciences, Grand Forks, North Dakota

HEATHER TRUDEAU, MPAS, PA-C
Preclinical Coordinator, Assistant Professor, Department of PA Medicine, Michigan State University College of Osteopathic Medicine, East Lansing, Michigan

ROGER D. WELLS, PA-C
Lexington Regional Health Center, Lexington, Nebraska

ANNE WILDERMUTH, MMS, PA-C, EM CAQ, RD
Assistant Professor, Associate Program Director and Director of Didactic Education, Department of Physician Assistant Studies, The George Washington University School of Medicine and Health Sciences, Washington, DC

MATTHEW WRIGHT, MS, PA-C, RD
Lecturer, Rutgers University School of Health Professions, Physician Assistant Program, Piscataway, New Jersey

JENNIFER SIMMS ZORN, DMS, PA-C
Associate Professor, Medical Science and Physician Assistant Studies Department, Butler University, Indianapolis, Indiana

Contents

> Greater awareness through public health strategies has improved diabetes screening, leading to improvements in early identification of prediabetes in at-risk patient populations. Early identification provides the opportunity for patients to prevent the progression of disease. Almost 20 years after the completion of the Diabetes Prevention Study, providers continue to look for strategies to help patients lose weight and increase physical activity levels to help prevent the progression from prediabetes to diabetes. Effective strategies for weight management for patients with prediabetes remains challenging and elusive to many clinicians. Clinicians can provide focused guidance and counseling through self-monitoring behaviors.

> Patients with diabetes are susceptible to complications, both microvascular (neuropathy) and macrovascular (peripheral arterial disease). Neuropathy can lead to loss of sensation and bony deformations. Peripheral arterial disease (PAD) can decrease blood flow and lead to lower extremity ischemia. Neuropathy, PAD and trauma from bony deformities increase the risk of foot ulceration and possible amputation. Regular comprehensive foot examinations allow providers to identify at-risk feet and recommend appropriate intervention to prevent complication development. This, combined with addressing modifiable risk factors like glycemic control, exercise, smoking cessation and home foot care help protect patients from developing foot ulcers, subsequent infections, amputations and early death.

> In the United States, cardiovascular disease (CVD) is the leading cause of death for men, women, and nearly every racial and ethnic group, with 655,000 deaths per year. Hypertension, hyperlipidemia, and tobacco abuse are key risk factors for CVD. Diabetes history, obesity, poor diet, physical inactivity, and excessive alcohol use are other factors. Adjuncts such as low-dose aspirin, fish oil supplements, and CT calcium scoring

organizational efforts focused on clinician well-being are paramount. PAs, as health care leaders, pave the way for wellness by identifying process areas that may cause an undue burden on health care providers, and encouraging psychological safety, open communication, and elimination of the mental health stigma.

Community Health

A community's resources and infrastructure impact the health and disease of individual members, but attention to the health of the community as a whole elevates the entire community. Communities that focus on public health can reduce inequality and reduce health disparities from race or ethnicity, social status, income, and any other issues discovered in this community. As physician assistants, we are often the bridge between our patients and community services. This article provides information and resources about clean water, healthy food, importance of physical activity, community safety, community education, social cohesion in a community, and health care access.

Sexual health is crucial to physical, emotional, and mental health that spans the individual, their partners, and their families. Sexual health-related issues vary and include sexual orientation, gender identity, sexual expression, relationships, and pleasure. Sexual health, if communicated with a positive, respectful, and informative approach with patients, can lead to an improvement in the patient's overall health and well-being. Therefore, there are measures as a health care provider that we can provide to cultivate an affirmative approach for sexual health with our patients, that is, through screening, vaccinations, and counseling.

This review of vaccines seeks to present topics for health care providers that will create optimal vaccination status in our patient populations. It will reinforce the pathophysiology and pharmacology of vaccines, as well as summarize current clinical guidelines for vaccine administration. The article describes some of the many barriers or limitations, cited by patients and parents and even some providers, to vaccine uptake. Finally, it will discuss strategies to improve provider vaccination literacy, methods for effective patient-provider dialogue, and ideas for improving vaccine uptake at the community level.

Health care disparities exist in many different entities including, but not limited to, age, race, ethnicity, gender identity, sexual orientation, socioeconomic status, technology, and access to care. Additional disparities include both mental and physical disabilities. This article dives in and explores many challenges that are faced by groups and individuals and identify areas of improvement as well as the areas of continued struggles, which calls for ongoing improvement.

Preventive health care for rural populations is challenged by provider scarcity, distance to care, transportation issues, and other social determinants of health. This article reviews the impact of those challenges.

Despite overall decreases in tobacco use over the past 50 years, the health consequences of smoking continue to be a significant issue for patients and clinicians. Although prevention measures are important, clinicians must also focus attention on identifying smokers through routine screening. There are a number of pharmacologic and nonpharmacologic treatments that can be use as smoking cessation measures and, when combined, their effectiveness increases.

Public health nutrition policy is shaped by nutritional epidemiologic studies, which inform medical society and association guidelines. These guidelines can help improve outcomes, decrease disease burden, and prevent morbidity and mortality; thus physician assistants should use these guidelines tailored to specific patient populations for nutrition recommendations.

The year 2020 will forever be associated with a new chapter in the history of global health, COVID-19. However, this new chapter would have a similar message because many other chapters were written before it. The COVID-19 pandemic would disproportionately affect minorities, those of low socioeconomic class, and those with limited access to health care. However, COVID-19 would also bring about a new health care disparity, limiting access to medical care for those with non COVID-19 related medical needs.

PHYSICIAN ASSISTANT CLINICS

SERIES OF RELATED INTEREST

Medical Clinics
https://www.medical.theclinics.com/
Primary Care: Clinics in Office Practice
https://www.primarycare.theclinics.com/

THE CLINICS ARE AVAILABLE ONLINE!
Access your subscription at:
www.theclinics.com

Foreword

Physician Assistants and Prevention Medicine

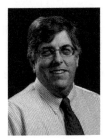

James A. Van Rhee, MS, PA-C
Consulting Editor

Physician assistants, disease prevention, and patient education have been linked since the beginning of the profession. From the first issue of the *Essentials of an Accredited Educational Program for the Assistant to the Primary Care Physician*, which stated the physician assistant's services would include, but not be limited to, the following: "instruction and counseling of patients regarding physical and mental health on matters such as diets, disease, therapy, and normal growth and development".[1] The current fifth issue of the *Accreditation Standards for Physician Assistant Education* states the curriculum must include instruction in patient education and referral, preventive patient encounters, and basic counseling and patient education skills.[2] So, preventive medicine has been one of the cores of physician assistant education since the beginning. In clinical practice, disease prevention and patient education are core competencies of the physician assistant profession. Preventive medicine plays a role in each physician assistant's clinical practice regardless of their specialty area of practice.

Because disease prevention and patient education play such an important role in physician assistant practice, this issue is past due as a topic in *Physician Assistant Clinics*. This issue, with guest editor, Stephanie Neary, provides an excellent review of several areas related to preventive medicine. We have divided these articles into three groups: those that cover clinical medicine, articles related to community health, and articles related to population health.

In clinical medicine topics, Kelly provides a discussion on diabetes prevention with a focus on lifestyle and behavior change. Lyon looks at ulcer prevention; Kilstrom and Wildermuth update us on cardiovascular disease prevention, and Jalaba, Trudeau, and Carlson look at obesity prevention. Kabara discusses optimizing the well-child check for children ages 3 to 18, while Hogg discusses preventive medicine in older

Physician Assist Clin 7 (2022) xv–xvi
https://doi.org/10.1016/j.cpha.2021.09.002
2405-7991/22/© 2021 Published by Elsevier Inc.

adults. Hoover and Bernard provide us with a call to action in regard to physician assistant well-being strategies.

Topics related to community health covered in this issue include Richardson and Dubé taking a physician assistant's perspective of health communities. Hopkins, Douglas, and Ady review various areas of sexual health preventive services. Chastain, Rippe, Solh, and Zorn look at vaccines, a hot topic of discussion around the globe currently. Regan, Lamb, and Early look at health disparities and access to care. Collett, Miller, and Wells discuss the challenges related to providing preventive health care in rural areas. Extending to population health, Ferschke describes the prevention and treatment of tobacco use. McReynolds, Park, and Wright discuss nutrition food policy guidelines. This issue finishes off with a very current topic, COVID-19 and health care inequality and disparity, discussed by Pieper.

I hope you enjoy this issue. Our next issue will cover topics related to the kidney.

James A. Van Rhee, MS, PA-C
Yale School of Medicine
Yale Physician Assistant Online Program
100 Church Street South, Suite A230
New Haven, CT 06519, USA

E-mail address:
james.vanrhee@yale.edu
Web Site:
www.paonline.yale.edu

REFERENCES

1. Sadler AM, Sadler BL, Bliss AA. Essentials of an approved educational program for the assistant to the primary care physician. The physician assistant: today and tomorrow. 2nd edition. Cambridge: Ballinger Publishing; 1975. p. 25–33.
2. Accreditation Review Commission on Education for the Physician Assistant. Accreditation standards for physician assistant education. 5th edition. Johns Creek, GA: ARC-PA; 2019. Available at: http://www.arc-pa.org/wp-content/uploads/2021/03/Standards-5th-Ed-March-2021.pdf. Accessed September 13, 2021.

Preface

Preventative Medicine

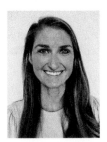

Stephanie L. Neary, MPA, MMS, PA-C
Editor

As physician assistants (PAs), we see patients who typically come to us when they need medical attention, not when they want to discuss preventing disease onset or progression. Through training, we focus on the pathophysiology, physical examination, diagnostics, and treatment of each condition discussed, but at what point do we expand this approach to also focus on prevention? While preventative health topics are added into curricula in various locations, why is this not a foundational concept we teach related to all conditions? This publication is by no means comprehensive; however, it seeks to bring forth awareness and knowledge surrounding common preventative health topics that are often overlooked.

Prevention can happen at many levels of the health care system; to mimic this, the preventive medicine topics presented here are grouped into three categories, including prevention at the individual level, prevention at the community level, and prevention at the national level. While there are many preventive health actions we can implement fairly easily into our own practices at the individual level, we should also be advocating for change in our communities and across the health care system as a whole. These larger systematic changes have the ability to change policy and improve access to care, but we can start with the patients we treat every day. There are times when we can push to change the system, but for many of us, we can make a much larger and sustained impact on the health of our patients by implementing preventative health discussions into our daily routines.

Many thanks to the collaborating providers for this issue of *Physician Assistant Clinics*, who are working tirelessly to serve their own communities. We can write about

Physician Assist Clin 7 (2022) xvii–xviii
https://doi.org/10.1016/j.cpha.2021.09.001
2405-7991/22/© 2021 Published by Elsevier Inc.

physicianassistant.theclinics.com

prevention all day, but it takes dedicated providers who are willing to modify their practice to create lasting change.

Stephanie L. Neary, MPA, MMS, PA-C
Yale Physician Assistant Online Program
PO Box 208004
New Haven, CT 06520-8004, USA

E-mail address:
stephanie.neary@yale.edu

Clinical Medicine

Diabetes Prevention
Focusing on Lifestyle and Behavior Change

Sarah Dion Kelly, MMSc, PA-C, RDN, CDCES

KEYWORDS

- Type 2 diabetes • Prediabetes • Self-monitoring • Diabetes prevention
- Weight management

KEY POINTS

- The progression of prediabetes to diabetes can be reduced with lifestyle changes that focus on moderate weight loss and increased physical activity.
- Lifestyle and behavior changes highlighted in the Diabetes Prevention Program offer simple, effective strategies for patients to lose weight and increase physical activity and maintain these behaviors over time.
- Pharmacologic options for weight loss continue to serve as adjunct therapies to lifestyle and behavior modification.

INTRODUCTION

Prediabetes was first described in 1965 by the World Health Organization (WHO), using the term "borderline diabetes."[1] Prediabetes was formally identified in 1999 by WHO by identifying a state of "intermediate hyperglycemia"[2] marked by both impaired glucose tolerance and fasting glucose. Type 2 diabetes (T2DM) is well known as a complex metabolic disease that develops over time. The pathophysiology of prediabetes and T2DM include the development of insulin resistance and pancreatic beta cell dysfunction. These 2 hallmark features occur along a spectrum of interrelated deficits of glucose metabolism. Diabetes develops when frank hyperglycemia results from pancreatic cell failure.[3] Prediabetes represents a timeline of hormonal dysregulation influenced by genetic and environmental factors. Environmental and lifestyle influences that are linked to the development of diabetes include but are not limited to age, sex, dietary intake, obesity, physical inactivity, socioeconomic status, and stress level.[4] The time leading up to diagnosis of T2DM is often marked by no overt symptoms; however, chronic inflammation and hyperinsulinemia are linked to the development of microvascular complications, such as cardiovascular disease[5] and retinopathy.[6] Incremental increases in 2-hour post-prandial blood glucoses are associated with the development of cardiovascular disease.[7] Fifty percent of patients with

Inova Cares Clinic for Families, 46440 Bendict Drive, Suite 208, Sterling, VA 20164, USA
E-mail address: Sarah.kelly@inova.org

Physician Assist Clin 7 (2022) 1–12
https://doi.org/10.1016/j.cpha.2021.08.012
2405-7991/22/© 2021 Elsevier Inc. All rights reserved.

prediabetes have been estimated to develop diabetes within 5 years of diagnosis.[2] In addition, those with gestational diabetes (GDM) also carry elevated risk of the development of T2DM in the future.

PREVALENCE AND ECONOMIC BURDEN

The global prevalence of diabetes among adults increased from 4.7% in 1980 to 8.5% in 2014 and the number of people with diabetes was estimated at 422 million in 2014.[8] Roughly 10% of the US population, or 34 billion, is estimated to have diabetes, with an estimated 20% being undiagnosed. Approximately one-third of the US population is estimated to have prediabetes, or roughly 88 million people. This percentage has stayed relatively stable between 2005 and 2016.[9] The total estimated financial burden of diabetes to US health care was estimated to be greater than $300 billion in 2017.[10] These statistics continue to support the importance of early detection of prediabetes with the goal of prevention or delay of progression to T2DM through lifestyle change.

RISK FACTORS, SCREENING AND DIAGNOSIS OF PREDIABETES/TYPE 2 DIABETES MELLITUS

Risk factors and screening guidelines have been outlined by the Centers for Disease Control and Prevention (CDC), American Diabetes Association, and US Preventive Services Task Force for prediabetes (**Boxes 1–3**). There are often no clear symptoms to prediabetes, so screening at-risk patients is paramount. The CDC has created a risk test that identifies people with a score of 10 or more to be at risk for T2DM (**Fig. 1**). The diagnosis of prediabetes and diabetes can be established through fasting plasma glucose (100–125 mg/dL), hemoglobin A1c (5.7%–6.4%), or oral glucose tolerance test (OGTT) (140–199 mg/dL).[3] See **Table 1** for diagnostic criteria.

Risk factors for diabetes-related complications are identified in the CDC National Diabetes Statistics Report. Smoking, overweight and obesity, physical inactivity, elevated HbA1C, elevated blood pressure, and elevated cholesterol were more common among those with diagnosed diabetes.[9] People with human immunodeficiency virus (HIV), including those on antiretroviral therapy, have higher prevalence of obesity, dyslipidemia, and T2DM.[11] Therefore, people with HIV should be screened regularly for T2DM.[3]

The increasing trends in obesity prevalence among youth highlight the need to screen children for prediabetes and T2DM.[12] Between 2015 and 2016, an estimated

---

Box 1
Centers for Disease Control and Prevention risk factors for prediabetes in adults[14]

Body mass index (BMI) greater than 25 (>23 in those that self-identify as Asian)

Age older than 45 years

Having a parent, brother, or sister with type 2 diabetes

Ever having gestational diabetes (diabetes during pregnancy)

Giving birth to a infant who weighed more than 9 pounds

Having polycystic ovary syndrome

Having nonalcoholic fatty liver disease

Certain race and ethnic groups are at higher risk: African American, Hispanic/Latino American, American Indian, Pacific Islander, and Asian American individuals.

Box 2
American Diabetes Association criteria for testing for diabetes or prediabetes in asymptomatic adults[3]

Adults with overweight or obesity (BMI $\geq$25 kg/m² or 23 kg/m² in Asian American individuals) and who have 1 or more of the following risk factors:
- First-degree relatives with diabetes
- High-risk race/ethnicity (African American, Latino, Native American, Asian American, Pacific Islander)
- History of cardiovascular disease
- Hypertension ($\geq$140/90 or on therapy for hypertension)
- High-density lipoprotein cholesterol level less than 35 mg/dL and/or a triglyceride level greater than 250 mg/dL
- Women with polycystic ovary syndrome
- Other clinical conditions associated with insulin resistance (severe obesity, acanthosis nigricans)

Patients with prediabetes (A1C greater than or equal to 5.7%) should be tested yearly

Women who were diagnosed with gestational diabetes should have lifelong testing every 3 years

For all other patients, testing should begin at age 45 years

If results are normal, testing should be repeated at a minimum of 3-year intervals, with consideration of more frequent testing depending on initial results and risk status

Human immunodeficiency virus

18.5% of children and adolescents ages 2 to 19 were obese, increasing from 13.5% in 1999 to 2000.[12] Screening for diabetes is recommended in youth who have a body mass index (BMI) greater than the 85th percentile (overweight), with a BMI of greater than the 95th percentile being classified as obese, and have one more additional risk factor (**Box 4**).[10] Pediatric obesity is a complex public health issue with genetic, environmental, socioeconomic, and behavioral influences. Clinicians and researchers alike continue to look for effective strategies to address its multifactorial etiology. Interventions that focus on dietary change, increased physical activity, eating behavioral modification, and the inclusion of family/caretakers have been shown to be effective.[13]

BEHAVIOR AND LIFESTYLE MODIFICATION

Intervention studies from around the globe have consistently supported the now well-accepted concept that moderate weight loss (less than 10% of starting body weight) and increased physical activity can reduce the risk of developing diabetes. Although the concepts appear straightforward, patients struggle to attain and maintain weight loss. Clinicians also struggle to provide effective guidance and support. Changing dietary and physical activity habits proves to be challenging and requires sustained

Box 3
US Preventive Services Task Force Diabetes Screening Guidelines[15]

Adults aged 40 to 70 years who are overweight or obese
- Screen for abnormal blood glucose
- Offer or refer patients with abnormal blood glucose to intensive behavioral counseling interventions to promote a healthful diet and physical activity

Prediabetes Risk Test

1. How old are you?

Write your score in the boxes below

Younger than 40 years (0 points)
40–49 y (1 point)
50–59 y (2 points)
60 years or older (3 points)

2. Are you a man or a woman?

Man (1 point)   Woman (0 points)

3. If you are a woman, have you ever been diagnosed with gestational diabetes?

Yes (1 point)   No (0 points)

4. Do you have a mother, father, sister, or brother with diabetes?

Yes (1 point)   No (0 points)

5. Have you ever been diagnosed with high blood pressure?

Yes (1 point)   No (0 points)

6. Are you physically active?

Yes (0 points)   No (1 point)

7. What is your weight category?

(See chart at right)

Total score:

Height	Weight (lbs.)		
4'10"	119–142	143–190	191+
4'11"	124–147	148–197	198+
5'0"	128–152	153–203	204+
5'1"	132–157	158–210	211+
5'2"	136–163	164–217	218+
5'3"	141–168	169–224	225+
5'4"	145–173	174–231	232+
5'5"	150–179	180–239	240+
5'6"	155–185	186–246	247+
5'7"	159–190	191–254	255+
5'8"	164–196	197–261	262+
5'9"	169–202	203–269	270+
5'10"	174–208	209–277	278+
5'11"	179–214	215–285	286+
6'0"	184–220	221–293	294+
6'1"	189–226	227–301	302+
6'2"	194–232	233–310	311+
6'3"	200–239	240–318	319+
6'4"	205–245	246–327	328+
	1 Point	**2 Points**	**3 Points**

You weigh less than the 1 Point column (0 points)

Adapted from Bang et al., Ann Intern Med 151:775-783, 2009. Original algorithm was validated without gestational diabetes as part of the model.

If you scored 5 or higher

You are at increased risk for having prediabetes and are at high risk for type 2 diabetes. However, only your doctor can tell for sure if you have type 2 diabetes or prediabetes, a condition in which blood sugar levels are higher than normal but not high enough yet to be diagnosed as type 2 diabetes. **Talk to your doctor to see if additional testing is needed.**

If you are African American, Hispanic/Latino American, American Indian/Alaska Native, Asian American, or Pacific Islander, you are at higher risk for prediabetes and type 2 diabetes. Also, if you are Asian American, you are at increased risk for type 2 diabetes at a lower weight (about 15 pounds lower than weights in the 1 Point column). Talk to your doctor to see if you should have your blood sugar tested.

You can reduce your risk for type 2 diabetes

Find out how you can reverse prediabetes and prevent or delay type 2 diabetes through a **CDC-recognized lifestyle change program** at https://www.cdc.gov/diabetes/prevention/lifestyle-program.

Fig. 1. The CDC Prediabetes Risk Test is a tool to identify those at risk for prediabetes. (Prediabetes Risk Test. accessed 7/19/2021 https://www.cdc.gov/diabetes/prevention/pdf/Prediabetes-Risk-Test-Final.pdf)

effort, through self-monitoring behaviors. The dietary and other lifestyle behaviors associated with overweight and obesity have been compared with those who struggle with addiction, and require frequent follow-up, counseling, support, and guidance.[16] A multitude of lifestyle intervention studies have provided support to long-term behavior modification programs that provide frequent contact, reinforcement of strategies, and individual and/or group support.

One of the earliest studies was the Da-Qing Diabetes Prevention Study, a lifestyle intervention study in Chinese community health clinics that began recruitment in

Table 1
Prediabetes and diabetes diagnostic criteria[3]

Test	Prediabetes	Diabetes
A1C	5.7%–6.4%	$\geq$6.5%
FPG	100–125 mg/dL	$\geq$126 mg/dL
OGTT	140–199 mg/dL	$\geq$200 mg/dL
RPG		$\geq$200 mg/dL

Abbreviations: A1C, Hemoglobin A1c, glycated hemoglobin; FPG, fasting plasma glucose; OGTT, oral glucose tolerance test; RPG, random plasma glucose.

1986. A total of 576 participants with impaired glucose tolerance were assigned to different programs of dietary intervention, physical activity, or both. The initial follow-up of these cohorts continued over a subsequent 6-year period. Dietary counseling focused on increasing vegetable intake, decreasing alcohol and refined carbohydrates, as well as reduced calorie intake. Participants in the physical activity intervention were instructed to engage in 20 minutes of brisk walking daily. The cumulative incidence of diabetes in the control group was 67% compared with 43.8%, 41.1%, and 46.0% in the intervention groups (diet only, exercise only, and diet and exercise groups, respectively).[17] After 30 years of follow-up, 540 participants from the original intervention were assessed for morbidity and mortality outcomes.[18] Compared with the control, the combined intervention groups saw delayed onset of diabetes (3.96 years) as well as fewer cardiovascular events, cardiovascular deaths, and microvascular complications, as well as increased life expectancy.[17]

The Finnish Diabetes Prevention Study was a randomized, multisite intervention study from 1993 to 2000. Roughly 500 overweight, middle-aged adults with impaired glucose tolerance among 5 different Finnish cities were randomized to an intensive lifestyle intervention or conventional therapy.[19] The intensive lifestyle intervention included individualized dietary and physical activity counseling as well as opportunities for circuit-type resistance training. The conventional therapy group received general dietary and exercise advice at baseline and then had annual physician examinations. The intensive lifestyle intervention group saw greater weight loss than the conventional group at 1 year (4.5 kg) and at 3 years (3.5 kg) compared with the conventional group (1.0 kg and 0.9 kg). Some key features of the intervention included face-to-face consultation sessions with a nutritionist with pre-planned topics including problem solving, nutritional guidance on saturated fat and fiber, physical activity, and

Box 4
Screening for diabetes in youth[10]

BMI greater than 85th percentile and 1 or more of the following risk factors:
1. Maternal history of diabetes or gestational diabetes during the child's gestation
    a. Family history of type 2 diabetes in first-degree or second-degree relatives
    b. Race/ethnicity (Native American, Africa American, Latino, Asian American, Pacific Islander)
    c. Signs of insulin resistance or conditions associated with insulin resistance
    d. Acanthosis nigricans
    e. Hypertension
    f. Dyslipidemia
    g. Polycystic ovary syndrome
    h. Small for gestational age birth weight

diabetes risk factors. These discussions were individualized to the participant. The Finnish Diabetes Prevention Study extended follow-up study over 7 years showed a 46% risk reduction in the development of diabetes.[20]

The Diabetes Prevention Study was a US-based multisite randomized intervention including 27 centers and approximately 1000 participants with an average of 2.8 years of follow-up. Participants were randomized to 1 of 3 interventions: (1) standard lifestyle intervention + metformin 850 mg twice daily, (2) standard lifestyle intervention + placebo, or (3) intensive lifestyle modification.[21] The intensive lifestyle intervention included outcome goals of 7% weight loss and 150 minutes of physical activity per week. Results of the study showed that the intensive lifestyle intervention group was more effective than metformin alone. Among the lifestyle modification group, a 58% reduction in incidence of T2DM was observed. Among the metformin group a 31% reduction in T2DM was observed. Key features of the lifestyle modification group included the use of trained lifestyle coaches, frequent contact with participants, a curriculum that focused on behavioral self-management strategies for weight loss and physical activity, and individuation through a toolbox of adherence strategies.[21] In subsequent follow-up evaluations, lifestyle intervention continued to support at least 34% reduction in diabetes incidence at 10 years and 17% reduction in diabetes incidence at 15 years.[22,23]

The Diabetes Prevention Program Study paved the way for the design and implementation of the CDC National Diabetes Prevention Program (DPP).[24] This program is a community-based lifestyle intervention program for people with and at risk for prediabetes. More than 1500 diabetes prevention programs exist throughout all 50 United States and several US territories.[25] These programs operate in a variety of settings ranging from community centers such as local YMCA groups and church organizations, as well as hospital-based programs. Medicare now provides reimbursement for participants that satisfactorily complete a CDC-recognized DPP. To qualify for enrollment in a DPP, participants need to have a BMI greater than 24 (or >22 if self-identified as Asian) and either have a score of 10 or more on the CDC prediabetes risk test (see **Fig. 1**) or 1 of the following: (1) have a personal history of gestational diabetes, (2) have a diagnosis of prediabetes through HbA1C test, fasting blood glucose, or OGTT. The program goals for participants include weight loss of 5% to 7% of initial body weight and attaining 150 minutes of moderate intensity physical activity per week. Participants meet in groups led by trained lifestyle coaches weekly for 24 sessions over the first 6 months, followed by monthly sessions for the maintenance period of the program (second 6 months of the program). Some hallmark features of these sessions include group education and support on nutrition, cooking, shopping, physical activity, stress management, goal setting, and sleep, as well as cardiovascular disease risk factors, specifically, blood pressure, cholesterol levels, and smoking cessation. There is reinforcement of self-monitoring behaviors through weigh-ins, tracking food and fitness. Participants are educated and encouraged to lose weight at a rate of no more than 1 to 2 pounds per week. Participants must weigh on a scale weekly and report their weight to the lifestyle coach. Participants are expected to track and report their fitness minutes weekly. The goal is to accumulate 150 minutes of moderate intensity activity per week (such as brisk walking). Throughout the program, participants are encouraged to track their food intake and submit it to the lifestyle coach for feedback. In total, the year-long behavior change program consists of 26 group support sessions occurring over 12 months. Some basic strategies that are reinforced throughout the program include decreasing total calorie intake by 500 to 1000 calories daily to create energy deficit, tracking food intake on a food log, increase fruit and vegetable intake, focus on portion control of carbohydrates and proteins, and choose

Box 5
"OARS": key elements of motivational interviewing[29]

Key Elements of Motivational Interviewing: OARS
  O: Ask open-ended questions
  A: Affirm the patient's perspective
  R: Reflect what was heard to ensure understanding
  S: Summarize shared understanding to set specific goals

healthy fats to incorporate into cooking. Lifestyle coaches provide focused guidance on exercise frequency, intensity type, and time. Other behavioral strategies include eating meals on a schedule, eating breakfast daily, and drinking water and other calorie-free beverages.[26]

The National Weight Control Registry is a large database of individuals who have successfully lost at least 30 pounds and maintained that weight loss for more than 1 year.[27] Members of this registry have lost on average 33 kg and maintained it for more than 5 years. Successful behavior strategies that were consistently reported among participants included self-monitoring of body weight, eating breakfast regularly, high levels of physical activity (approximately 1 hour per day), eating regular meals, and eating a low-calorie, low-fat diet.[27] Self-monitoring, or "tracking," behaviors help to provide patients with the daily feedback needed to reinforce healthy eating and physical activity habits.

When possible, clinicians should refer patients with prediabetes for medical nutrition therapy counseling with a registered dietitian-nutritionist (RDN). Medical nutrition therapy (MNT) consists of nutrition assessment, diagnosis, intervention, and management to create an individualized food plan with support and follow-up. The RDN provides individualized meal planning and hands-on strategies to change eating habits. The MNT incorporates cultural and personal preferences. For adults with T2DM, MNT has been demonstrated to reduce hemoglobin A1 by 0.3% to 2%.[28] MNT is a covered benefit provided by most commercial insurance and typically consists of a series of 3 or more encounters lasting 45 to 90 minutes each.

Motivational interviewing (MI) is an effective tool that clinicians can use to facilitate weight management as well as other health-related behavior change. This method of counseling allows the patient to lead the path and define the outcome of the encounter. MI includes important principles of empathy, discrepancy, and

Box 6
Tips for motivational interviewing

1. Determine the patient's desire for change. "On a scale of 1 to 10, how important is achieving a healthy weight status as goal for you?"
   • Determine patient confidence in their ability to make the change. "On a scale of 1 to 10, how confident are you that you can make the necessary changes to achieve a healthy weight status?"
   • Obtain a commitment (verbally or, preferably, in writing) to making the necessary changes.
   • Do not oppose a patient if they are resistant to change ("roll with resistance").
   • Summarize the patient's "change talk" as part of a patient-centered dialogue.
   • Create a patient-directed plan for making necessary changes.

Reprinted with permission Kelly CP, Sbrocco G, Sbrocco T. Behavioral Modification for the management of obesity. *Primary Care.* 2016. 43(1):159 to 175.

Table 2
Medications for weight management[2]

Name	Dose	Mechanism of Action	Mean Percent Weight Loss	Side Effects
Orlistat	120 mg 3 times daily	Pancreatic lipase inhibitor	−6.1%	Cramping, increased defecation, anal leakage, flatus.
Liraglutide	3.0 mg injection daily[a]	GLP-1 receptor agonist	−7.4%	Nausea, diarrhea, headache.
Phentermine/ Topiramate Extended Release	7.5 mg/46 mg 15 mg/92 mg[a]	Sympathomimetic Anticonvulsant	−7.8%	Paresthesia, dizziness, dysgeusia, insomnia, constipation, and dry mouth.
Naltrexone Sustained Release (SR)/ Bupropion SR	32 mg/360 mg[a]	Opioid receptor antagonist Dopamine and noradrenaline reuptake inhibitor	−5.4%	Nausea, constipation, headache, vomiting, dizziness, insomnia, dry mouth, and diarrhea.

[a] These medications require dose titration.

identification of resistance.[29] It is focused on exploring and resolving ambivalence as well as facilitating self-efficacy. Key techniques of MI include open-ended questions, reflective listening and statements, and the facilitation of "change talk" (**Box 5**). Ultimately, the goal as the provider is to facilitate relative and attainable goal setting, for those patients who are ready for change. Using concepts from the transtheoretical model of behavioral change, clinicians can help patients identify precontemplation, contemplation, preparation, action, maintenance, and/or relapse phases.[30] A systematic review of the use of MI for weight loss in primary care supported potential benefits for patients.[31]

PHARMACOLOGIC THERAPY AND BARIATRIC SURGERY

Metformin is effective in the prevention of T2DM.[32] The Diabetes Prevention Study demonstrated a 31% risk reduction in the development of T2DM in the metformin alone group. Another meta-analysis of 3 lifestyle intervention studies for diabetes prevention estimated a 4% to 14% risk reduction in diabetes with metformin use alone.[33] Metformin has been demonstrated to be cost-effective and potentially cost-saving.[32] Metformin may reduce the risk of cardiovascular disease and death.[23] A biguanide drug, its primary mechanisms aim to reduce hepatic glucose production, fasting, and postprandial hyperglycemia and improve peripheral insulin sensitivity.[34] Metformin has a side effect of weight loss and has been shown to induce significant weight loss in obese individuals without diabetes.[35] Metformin therapy should be considered for those with prediabetes, particularly those with a hemoglobin A1C in the upper end of the prediabetes range of 6.0% to 6.4%.[32] Main side effects with initiation include gastrointestinal side effects of bloating, abdominal discomfort, and diarrhea, but these can be mitigated by slow initiation and titration. Metformin is contraindicated in patients with an estimated glomerular filtration rate $\geq$30 mL/min per 1.73 m^2.[36]

Other pharmacologic strategies can serve as adjunct therapy to diet, exercise, and behavioral interventions for weight loss and/or weight loss maintenance. Indications to add pharmacotherapy for the treatment of obesity include elevated BMI $\geq$27 with comorbid conditions or $\geq$30, or failure to achieve and/or sustain meaningful weight loss of greater than 5% of total body weight.[37–42] Current medications in use are summarized in **Box 6** and **Table 2** and include liraglutide, orlistat, phentermine-topiramate, and naltrexone-bupropion.

Last, bariatric surgery is an effective intervention strategy for those with morbid obesity. Bariatric surgery is indicated for those with BMI greater than 40 or greater than 35 with comorbid conditions. A variety of surgical options are now available (adjustable gastric banding, vertical sleeve gastrectomy, roux-en-Y gastric bypass and biliopancreatic diversion with or without duodenal switch). Weight loss after bariatric surgery is often measured in excess body weight loss and has been reported between 49% and 71%.[43] For those with T2DM before bariatric surgery, diabetes remission and reduced microvascular and macrovascular complications have been observed in long-term (>5 years) outcomes studies.[44] Patients typically have long-term success with sustained weight loss, and resolution of metabolic abnormalities such as prediabetes and diabetes has been reported. However, weight gain relapse and complications are reported.

SUMMARY

Important features of diabetes prevention include early identification and intervention to change lifestyle behaviors, with a focus on lifestyle change, eating habits, and increased physical activity. Screening for prediabetes and diabetes should be completed in those patients with risk factors. Individualized counseling using MI should be used to help patients address personal lifestyle habits. Referral to group-based community diabetes prevention programs will provide patients the support and follow-up they require for success. Pharmacologic and surgical therapy options continue to serve as adjunct to the mainstay of lifestyle change through improved eating habits and increased physical activity.

CLINICS CARE POINTS

- Prediabetes is often asymptomatic, so screening at-risk populations is paramount to early identification.
- Those with BMI greater than 25 and other risk factors should be screened regularly for prediabetes.
- Moderate weight loss of between 5% and 10% has positive effects on insulin resistance and diabetes disease progression in those with prediabetes.
- Self-monitoring behaviors such as tracking fitness, food, and body weight helps people lose weight and maintain the weight loss.
- MI is a tool that clinicians should learn and practice to help their patients tackle lifestyle change interventions.

DISCLOSURE

The author has nothing to disclose.

REFERENCES

1. Colagiuri S. Epidemiology of prediabetes. Med Clin North Am 2011;95:299–307.
2. Tabak AG, Herder C, Rathmann W, et al. Prediabetes: a high-risk state for developing diabetes. Lancet 2012;379(9833):2279–90.
3. American Diabetes Association. Classification and diagnosis of diabetes: standards of medical care in diabetes - 2021. Diabetes Care 2021;44(Suppl 1):S15–33.
4. Kautzy-Willer A, Harreiter J, Pacini G. Sex and gender differences in risk, pathophysiology and complications of type 2 diabetes mellitus. Endocr Rev 2016;34(3):278–316.
5. The Diabetes Prevention Program Research Group. Impact of intensive lifestyle and metformin therapy on cardiovascular disease risk factors in the diabetes prevention program. Diabetes Care 2005;28:888–94.
6. Lamparter J, Raum P, Pfeiffer N, et al. Prevalence and associations of diabetic retinopathy in a large cohort of prediabetic subjects: the Gutenberg Health Study. J Diabetes Complications 2014;28(4):482–7.
7. Meigs JB, Nathan DM, D'Agostina RB, et al. Fasting and postchallenge glycemia and cardiovascular disease risk. Diabetes Care 2002;25:1845–50.
8. Diabetes. Key facts. 2020. Available at: https://www.who.int/news-room/fact-sheets/detail/diabetes. Accessed November 24, 2020.
9. Center for Disease Control. National diabetes statistics report. 2020. Available at: https://www.cdc.gov/diabetes/pdfs/data/statistics/national-diabetes-statistics-report.pdf. Accessed January 25, 2021.
10. American Diabetes Association. Standards of medical care. Diabetes Care 2021;44(1):S7–39.

11. Monroe AK, Glesby MJ, Brown TT. Diagnosing and managing diabetes in HIV-Infected patients: current concepts. Clin Infect Dis 2014;60:453–62.

12. Hales CM, Carroll MD, Fryar CD, et al. Prevalence of obesity among adults and youth: United States, 2015–2016. NCHS Data Brief 2017;(288):1–8.

13. Snethen JA, Broome ME, Cashin SE. Effective weight loss for overweight children: a meta-analysis of intervention studies. J Pediatr Nurs 2006;21(1):45–56.

14. Centers for Disease Control. Diabetes risk factors. Available at: https://www.cdc.gov/diabetes/basics/risk-factors.html. Accessed January 25, 2021.

15. US Preventive Task Force. Abnormal blood glucose and type 2 diabetes: screening. 2015. Available at: https://www.uspreventiveservicestaskforce.org/uspstf/recommendation/screening-for-abnormal-blood-glucose-and-type-2-diabetes. Accessed January 25, 2021.

16. Armstrong MJ, Moltenshead TA, Ronksley PE, et al. Motivational interviewing to improve weight loss in overweight and/or obese patients: a systematic review and meta-analysis of randomized controlled trials. Obes Rev 2011;(12):709–23.

17. Pan XR, Li GW, Hu YH, et al. Effects of diet and exercise in preventing NIDDM in people with impaired glucose tolerance: the Da Qing IGT and diabetes Study. Diabetes Care 1997;(4):537–44.

18. Gong Q, Zhang P, Wang J, et al. Morbidity and mortality after lifestyle intervention for people with impaired glucose tolerance: 30-year results of the Da Qing Diabetes Prevention Outcome Study. Lancet Diabetes Endocrinol 2019;7:452–61.

19. Lindstrom J, Louheranta A, Mannelin M, et al. The Finnish diabetes prevention study. Diabetes Care 2003;26(12):3230–6.

20. Lindstrom J, Ilanne-Parikka P, Peltonen M, et al. Sustained reduction in the incidence of type 2 diabetes by lifestyle intervention: follow-up of the Finnish Diabetes Prevention Study. Lancet 2006;368:1673–9.

21. Diabetes Prevention Program Research Group. Reduction in the incidence of type 2 diabetes with lifestyle intervention or metformin. N Eng J Med 2002;346(6):393–406.

22. Diabetes Prevention Program Research Group. 10-year follow-up of diabetes incidence and weight loss in the Diabetes Prevention Program Outcomes Study. Lancet 2009;374(9702):1677–86.

23. Diabetes Prevention Program Research Group. Long-term effects of lifestyle intervention or metformin on diabetes development and microvascular complications; the DPP Outcomes Study. Lancet Diabetes Endocrinol 2015;3(11):866–975.

24. National diabetes prevention program. Available at: https://www.cdc.gov/diabetes/prevention/index.html. Accessed January 18, 2021.

25. National Diabetes Prevention Program. Registry of all recognized programs. Available at: https://www.nccd.cd.gov/DDT_DPRP/Registry.aspx. Accessed January 18.

26. National Diabetes Prevention Program. Curricula and handouts. Available at: https://www.cdc.gov/diabetes/prevention/resources/curriculum.html. Accessed January 25, 2021.

27. Wing RR, Phelan S. Long-term weight loss maintenance. Am J Clin Nutr 2005;82(suppl):222S–5S.

28. Briggs K, Stanley K. Position of the Academy of Nutrition and Dietetics: the role of medical nutrition therapy and registered dietitian nutritionists in the prevention and treatment of prediabetes and type 2 diabetes. J Acad Nutr Diet 2018;118:343–53.

29. Kelly CP, Sbrocco G, Sbrocco T. Behavioral modification for the management of obesity. Prim Care 2016;43(1):159–75.
30. Prochaska JO, Velicer WF. The transtheoretical model of health behavior change. Am J Health Promot 1997;12(1):38–48.
31. Barnes RD, Ivezaj V. A systematic review of motivational interviewing for weight loss among adults in primary care. Obes Rev 2015;16:304–18.
32. Moin T, Schmittdiel JA, Flory JH, et al. Review of metformin use for type 2 diabetes prevention. Am J Prev Med 2018;55(4):565–74.
33. Li CL, Pan CY, Lu JM, et al. Effect on metformin on patients with impaired glucose tolerance. Diabet Med 1999;16(6):477–81.
34. Gong L, Goswami S, Giacomini KM, et al. Metformin pathways: pharmacokinetics and pharmacodynamics. Pharmacogenet Genomics 2012;22(11):820–7.
35. Seifarth C, Schehler B, Schneider HJ. Effectiveness of metformin on weight loss in non-diabetic individuals with obesity. Exp Clin Endocrinol Diabetes 2013;121(1):27–31.
36. American Diabetes Association. Pharmacological approaches to glycemic treatment: standards of medical are in diabetes-2021. Diabetes Care 2021;44(Suppl. 1):S111–24.
37. Apovian CM, Aronne LJ, Bessesen DH, et al. Pharmacological management of obesity: an endocrine society clinical practice guideline. J Clin Endocrinol Metab 2015;100:342–62.
38. Highlights of prescribing information. Xenical® (orlistat). 2012. Available at: https://www.accessdata.fda.gov/drugsatfda_docs/label/2012/020766s029lbl.pdf. Accessed January 25, 2021.
39. Highlights of prescribing information. Victoza® (liraglutide). Available at: https://www.accessdata.fda.gov/drugsatfda_docs/label/2019/022341s031lbl.pdf. Accessed January 25, 2021.
40. Highlights of prescribing information. Belviq® (locaserin). Available at: https://www.accessdata.fda.gov/drugsatfda_docs/label/2012/022529lbl.pdf. Accessed January 25, 2021.
41. Highlights of prescribing information. Qsymia® (phentermine-topiramate ER). Available at: https://www.accessdata.fda.gov/drugsatfda_docs/label/2012/022580s000lbl.pdf. Accessed January 25, 2021.
42. Highlights of prescribing information. Contrave® (naltrexone-bupropion HCl ER). Available at: https://www.accessdata.fda.gov/drugsatfda_docs/label/2014/200063s000lbl.pdf. Accessed January 25, 2021.
43. O'Brien PE, Hindle A, Brennan L, et al. Long-term outcomes after bariatric surgery: a systematic review and meta-analysis of weight loss at 10 or more years for all bariatric procedures and a single-centre review of 20-year outcomes after adjustable gastric banding. Obes Surg 2019;29:3–14.
44. Sheng B, Truong K, Spitler H, et al. The long-term effects of bariatric surgery on type 2 diabetes remission, microvascular and macrovascular complications and mortality: a systematic review and meta-analysis. Obes Surg 2017;27:2724–32.

Diabetic Ulcer Prevention

Melanie M. Lyon, MSPAS, PA-C

KEYWORDS

- Diabetic ulcer • Neuropathy • Peripheral arterial disease • Diabetic foot examination
- Monofilament

KEY POINTS

- Diabetic foot ulcers are complications that occur secondary to vascular, neuropathic, and biomechanical changes and foot deformities.
- Prevention of diabetic foot complications includes identifying the at-risk foot with comprehensive, regular foot examinations, and referring for appropriate care.
- Screening for loss of protective sensation can be detected by using the nylon Semmes-Weinstein monofilament test.
- Assessment for peripheral arterial disease by measuring ankle-brachial index is another helpful screening test.
- Optimizing glycemic control, regular exercise, smoking cessation, and at-home foot examinations can help reduce the risk foot ulceration.

INTRODUCTION

According to the CDC & the National Diabetes Statistics Report, as of 2018 there are 34.2 million US adults with diabetes, a metabolic disorder characterized by hyperglycemia as a result of the body's dependence on exogenous insulin (type 1) or relative insulin deficiency and/or resistance (type 2). Patients with diabetes, especially those whose blood sugar levels remain poorly controlled, may develop one or many chronic complications that may impact multiple organ systems. These diabetic chronic complications can be grouped as either vascular or nonvascular. Vascular complications can further be grouped into microvascular and macrovascular (**Table 1**). Diabetic ulcers are lesions that involve a break in the skin with a loss of epithelium. They are most commonly found on the plantar surface of the foot and are often caused by a combination of both microvascular and macrovascular complications.[1] Depending on the severity of the ulcer, it may extend further into the dermis, muscle, and/or bone.

The incidence of diabetic foot ulcers (DFUs) is estimated to be between 19% and 34% in a diabetic's lifetime and the cost burden of diabetic foot disease is amongst the top 10 of all medical conditions.[2–4] Foot ulcers resulting from diabetes increase

Neighborhood Outreach Access to Health – HonorHealth, 9201 North 5th Street, Phoenix, AZ 85020, USA
E-mail address: mlyon@honorhealth.com

Physician Assist Clin 7 (2022) 13–29
https://doi.org/10.1016/j.cpha.2021.07.002
2405-7991/22/© 2021 Elsevier Inc. All rights reserved.

Table 1		
Chronic complications of diabetes and manifestations		
Vascular		Nonvascular
Microvascular	Macrovascular	

• Nephropathy
• Neuropathy
• Retinopathy
	• Cerebrovascular disease
	• Coronary arterial disease
	• Peripheral arterial disease
		• Cognitive impairment
		• Dermatologic
		  ○ Acanthosis nigricans
		  ○ Infections
		• Gastroparesis
		• Hearing loss
		• Ocular
		  ○ Cataracts
		  ○ Glaucoma
		• Periodontal disease
		• Sexual dysfunction

Data from Ref.[2]

the incidence of hospital admission 11-fold.[5] Although preventable, infected ulcers are the most common reason for hospital admission in the United States and in 2017 had a total direct and indirect estimated cost of $327 billion.[6]

In addition to the significant cost burden to the medical system, ulcers can lead to severe long-term complications and consequences including loss of limb and life. DFU and amputations are associated with a diminished quality of life at rates similar to that of patients with cancer. It can drastically worsen not just physical but also the psychological and social quality of life of those afflicted.[7,8] It is estimated that 85% of all amputations are preceded by an ulcer2, and the risk of amputation is between 10 and 20 times more likely for those with diabetes than without.[9] Even more alarming is the 5-year mortality rate following a lower limb amputation at more than 50%.[10]

The serious potential outcomes of DFUs cannot be underestimated and prevention of ulceration is essential. With a systematic and comprehensive approach to diabetic foot care, primary care providers can shift the focus to upstream interventions that can help prevent ulcer formation and subsequent decreased quality of life, amputation, and early death.

OVERVIEW: FACTORS THAT CONTRIBUTE TO ULCER FORMATION

DFUs are the result of the simultaneous actions of many causes. The most common known causes include neuropathy, deformity, and their resultant trauma[11] Once an ulcer develops, there are several factors that contribute to the adverse outcome of amputation. The most important of these is atherosclerotic peripheral vascular disease which particularly affects the femoropopliteal and smaller vessels below the knee.[12,13]

Preventing foot complications begins with identifying patients at risk. In addition to neuropathy, deformity and trauma, there are other important historical factors shown to contribute to the risk of ulcer formation. Patients with a history of foot ulcers, prior lower extremity amputations, and neuropathy have been shown to have the highest risk of ulceration and amputation.[12,14]

Other demonstrated risk factors to consider include impaired vision less than 20/40, length of diabetes diagnosis greater than 10 years, and elevated A1C >8.[12,13,15–18] Hyperglycemia and abnormal glucose metabolism are shown to increase the incidence of neuropathy and peripheral arterial disease (PAD), as well as the progression of the diseases and their severity.[19]

Table 2 provides the key elements to address in a patient's history and review of systems when assessing foot risk in patients with diabetes.[18] Identifying patients with at-risk feet can provide guidance to health care providers and patients to best prevent ulcer formation and its complications[20,21]

Health care providers should aim to screen for the following three relevant contributing factors to begin:

1. Vasculopathy
2. Neuropathy
3. Trauma

VASCULOPATHY
Peripheral Arterial Disease

PAD stems from atherosclerosis of the lower extremity arteries and results in the narrowing or occlusion of blood vessels. This leads to the lack of blood flow and development of lower extremity ischemia. The resultant restriction of oxygenated, nutrient-rich blood to the site of the ulcer increases the risk; it will become infected and heal slowly or worsen.[19,22] It may also negatively impact healing by disrupting the delivery of systemic antibiotics to infected wounds. PAD not only affects up to 50% of diabetics with ulcers but also results in worse lower extremity function when compared with patients without diabetes. Additionally, PAD is a known major risk factor of lower extremity amputation accelerated by the direct damage of nerves and blood vessels secondary to hyperglycemia.[14,19,23]

Screening for Peripheral Arterial Disease

The initial assessment of PAD should begin with a complete history and review of systems, including the factors show in **Table 2**. Clinical signs and symptoms of PAD vary on a wide spectrum. Some patients may be asymptomatic, whereas others may experience one or more of the following complaints: leg weakness, pain or cramping that occurs during activity and is improved with rest.[24] Asymptomatic patients or patients with neuropathy may not be aware that they have PAD or have more subtle signs. As a result, it is important for primary care providers to complete a thorough physical examination and assess their patients regularly to ensure early intervention or prevention of

Table 2		
Key elements of the history and review of systems diabetic foot risk		
Prior History	**Social History**	**Medical History**
• Ulcer	• Smoking	• Duration of Diabetes
• Amputation	• Socioeconomic Factors	• Hemoglobin A1C levels
	○ Finances (cost of medication, visits, devices, etc.)	• Impaired vision
	○ Education	• Kidney disease
	○ Access to services	
	○ Access to nutrition	
Vascular Symptoms	**Neuropathy Symptoms**	**Trauma Risk**
• Intermittent claudication	• Numbness	• History of foot surgery
• Pain at rest	• Tingling	• Activity level (exercise level, occupation)
• Nonhealing ulcer	• Pain (sharp, burning, electrical shocks, etc.)	

Data from Refs.[11,19]

PAD and consequential poor healing ulcers and infections. **Table 3** provides the key elements of the complete diabetic foot examination, including vascular assessment, for review.

Clinical evidence of PAD may include cool skin, nail thickening, lack of leg hair below the knee, thinning of skin on the legs, dependent rubor (red skin that blanches with elevation), cool, dry, fissured skin and/or diminished lower extremity pulses. The vascular physical assessment must include palpation of the posterior tibial and dorsalis pedis pulses and noted to be either present or absent.[11] The absence of both pedal pulses strongly suggests the presence of vascular disease and has shown a 4.72 relative risk of ulcer formation versus a normal examination, where all four pulses are palpable. Unfortunately, the presence of palpable pulses cannot absolutely exclude PAD and further assessment may be needed.[25–27]

Assessment for Peripheral Arterial Disease

Patients with diabetes whose history and physical examination reveal signs or symptoms of PAD and/or absent pulses should undergo further examination. Options include the ankle-brachial index (ABI), digital arterial systolic pressures (toe pressures), toe-brachial index, doppler ultrasound, vascular imaging, and transcutaneous oxygen tension (TcPO$_2$). The American Diabetes Association recommends patients requiring further evaluation for PAD undergo ABI testing. This test is low cost, simple, reproducible, and has a sensitivity of 95% and specificity of 99% in diagnosing PAD.[27,28] The ABI is calculated by determining the ratio of systolic blood pressure in the ankle to that in the brachial artery. An ABI value $\leq$ 0.90 is diagnostic of PAD and warrants referral to a vascular surgeon. It is important to note that ABI measurements may be falsely elevated in patients with diabetes. This may occur due to the presence of medical arterial calcinosis which allows arteries to be incompressible. If the ABI is >1.3 other methods, such as toe pressure or TcPO$_2$ can be used to confirm or rule out PAD.[27,29]

NEUROPATHY

Diabetic neuropathy is a microvascular complication of Diabetes Mellitus (DM) that can alter autonomic, motor, and/or sensory functions. **Table 4** reviews the function

Table 3
Key elements of the comprehensive diabetic foot examination and risk assessment

Vascular	Neurologic	Musculoskeletal	Dermatologic
Test for:	Test for:	Inspect for:	Inspect for:
• Pedal pulses	• Sensation: 10 g	• Muscle strength	• Skin changes
• ABI, if absent or suspected PAD	monofilament	• Muscle wasting	○ Color
	• Small fiber: temperature or pin-prick	• Joint stiffness	○ Pigmentation
		• Deformities	○ Texture
	• Vibration/Large fiber: 128-Hz tuning fork	○ Hammer toe	○ Thickness
		○ Bunion	○ Dryness
		○ Prominent metatarsal heads	○ Sweating
	○ Or VPT	○ Charcot foot	• Infection
	• Motor: ankle reflexes		○ Odor
			○ Peeling between toes
			○ Thickened or discolored toenails

Data from Refs.[11,61]

Table 4 Peripheral nerve functions and malfunction		
Nerve Type	Normal Function	Malfunction/Ulcer Formation Contribution
Motor	Voluntary movement: talking, walking	Atrophy/Weakness of the foot/joint → abnormal walking pattern → increased pressure on plantar portion of foot
Sensory	Feeling: touch, temperature, pain	Loss of sensation → increased risk of injury, unknown wound, increased trauma to site
Autonomic	Nonvoluntary activities: breathing, circulation, digestion, gland function	Reduced or absent sweating → dry, cracked skin, fissures → infection

Data from Ref.[30]

of each peripheral nerve type. It is estimated to affect nearly 50% of patients with DM in their lifetime[30] and leads to an increased risk for extremity injuries, infection, ulcers, and lower extremity amputation. A seven-fold higher risk of developing an ulcer has been reported in patients with diabetes with moderate to severe sensory loss.[1] Poor balance and instability from the atrophy of the small muscles in the foot can lead to rigid deformities causing pain or contributing to ulcer formation. The dysregulation of local perspiration can result in reduced sweating on the foot making the skin prone to develop cracks, fissures, or secondary infections.[10]

The most common of the neuropathies, diabetic peripheral neuropathy (DPN), is defined as "the presence of symptoms and/or signs of peripheral nerve dysfunction in people with diabetes after the exclusion of other causes."[31] DPN is not only the most common cause of foot ulceration but also the severe foot deformity Charcot neuroarthropathy (CN).[32,33] See **Table 5** for details about this severe and late complication.

Screening for Neuropathy

Neuropathy is a progressive process and can ultimately lead to the loss of protective sensation. Once sensation is lost, the foot is susceptible to accidental injuries and daily repetitive stress.[14]

According to the American Diabetes Association and other organizations, assessment for neuropathy should begin 5 years after the diagnosis of type 1 diabetes or at the time of diagnosis of type 2 diabetes using a thorough history and physical examination.[34]

Like PAD, the clinical presentation of neuropathy signs and symptoms can be varied. Common complaints may include tingling, burning, numbness, dry and cracked feet, difficulty with balance and/or lower extremity muscle weakness. With the progressive nature of neuropathy in mind, the clinicians' assessment of sensation should consider both small and large nerve fiber involvement. **Table 3** provides the key elements of the complete diabetic foot examination, including neuropathy assessment, for review. Pain is the primary symptom of DPN involving the small fibers. The pain may be described as burning, shooting, or electric shocks and can greatly impact a patient's ability to complete daily activities and reduce their overall quality of life.[31] Symptoms of DPN involving the large fibers may include numbness, tingling without pain, and/or poor balance. When screening for DPN, the most commonly used noninvasive methods include testing for protective sensation and vibration perception. These tests are instrumental in detecting those at risk of diabetic ulcers and its associated morbidity and mortality.[34]

Table 5
A closer look at Charcot Neuroarthropathy (CN)

CN affects the bones, joints and soft tissues of the foot and ankle. Uncontrolled inflammation triggered by multiple factors, such as neuropathy, trauma, and excessive osteoclastic activity, leads to various patterns of pathologic fractures, joint dislocation & the destruction of the pedal architecture. Suspect CN in a patient who:
- Has history or symptoms of neuropathy
- Presents with an acute red, hot, swollen, foot after no or minimal trauma

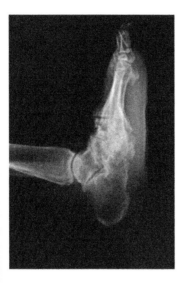

The hallmark deformity associated with CN is midfoot collapse and is often referred to as a "rocker-bottom" foot and represents a severe stage for this condition.

The diagnosis of active CN is primarily based on:
- History
- Clinical finding: inflammation is usually the earliest finding and can be confirmed by imaging.
- Plain radiographs should be initial choice.
- MRI or nuclear imaging can be used if XR are normal and clinical suspicion is high.

Management of CN includes:
- offloading the foot
- protective weight-bearing devices
- regular and lifetime surveillance
- +/− surgical treatment

Artwork from Porrini P. Royalty-Free Stock Photo ID: 1206902347. Accessed January 30, 2021. https://www.shutterstock.com/photos; Data from Refs.[32,33]

Health care providers should also examine the foot for muscle atrophy and deformities secondary to motor neuropathy and dry or thick skin secondary to autonomic neuropathy. Intrinsic muscle atrophy from motor neuropathy can weaken the digit stabilizers and progress to the ankle and knee. This weakness may result in overall gait instability, affecting the patient's ability to walk and lead to the development of foot deformities.[35,36] It is also important to examine the toenails and note any signs of infection, such as Onychomycosis and Tinea pedis. In the diabetic population, these common fungal infections may lead to a secondary systemic infection and increases the risk of an ulcer 3-fold.[37]

Assessment for Neuropathy

There are many clinical tests available to evaluate small- and large-fiber sensory function. The 5.07/10 g Semmes-Weinstein monofilament (SWMF) test has been a useful tool for detecting more advanced and large-fiber neuropathy, as well as those who may be at an increased risk of ulcer formation. It has been a preferred choice for screening and which is due to its low cost, portability, noninvasiveness, ease for patients and providers and sensitivity. Many studies have shown that when performed properly, health care providers can achieve up to 90% sensitivity and can predict the future of ulceration and likely lower extremity amputation for patients with diabetes.[38–40]

Recently, there has been some discrepancy in data regarding the sensitivity of the MF test to screen and monitor for the progression of DPN, supporting the current recommendation of using more than just the MF test alone during a neurologic examination.[41–43] In addition to the MF test, small-fiber function should be tested by either temperature sense or pin-prick test. Large-fiber function vibration sense should also be tested and can be completed using the 128-Hz tuning fork. An alternative test for vibration loss is the use of an electromechanical vibration perception threshold (VPT) meter, also known as, Biothesiometer or Neurothesiometer.[31]

The 5.07/10 g Semmes-Weinstein monofilament

The SWMF tests sensory neuropathy, specifically large fiber function, by exerting 10 g of pressure on the foot to test sensation.[25] With the patient's eyes closed, the tip of the fiber is placed on each of the preferred areas perpendicular to the foot until it buckles. Each time the patient feels the sensation they report with a verbal "yes." Traditionally, the test has been completed by using the 10 test sites shown in **Fig. 1** on each foot as follows: distal first toe, distal third toe, distal fifth toe, plantar first metatarsal head, plantar third metatarsal head, plantar fifth metatarsal head, plantar medial and lateral arch, plantar heel, and dorsal first interspace. In a recent study, there was no significant difference in the sensitivities of 3, 4, and 10 site SWMF testing.[44]

In 2017, the American Diabetes Association recommended that the screening should be completed on only four sites of each foot. The diagnosis of neuropathy is made if the patient fails to say yes at any of the four spots. It should also be noted that after numerous patient uses (10 or more) and without a recovery period of at least 24 before further use, the MF may buckle at a reduced amount of pressure leading to less accurate results.[45]

128-Hz tuning fork

With the patient's eyes closed and the feet on a flat surface, tap on the tuning fork. With the fork vibrating, place it on the patient's distal Hallux joint (dorsal side) and ask the patient if they can feel the sensation by answering yes or no. The test is noted to be positive when the patient loses vibratory sensation despite the examiners ability to still perceive it.[11,12]

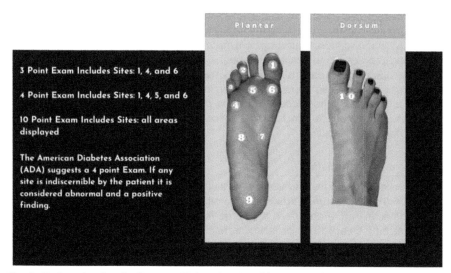

Fig. 1. Testing sites for the Semmes-Weinstein Monofilament Evaluation. (Artwork courtesy of Amber Price, PA-C; *Data from* Refs.[42–44].)

Vibration perception threshold meter

The VPT meter is held with a probe on or under the pulp of the toe. The examiner increases the voltage on the base until the patient perceives the vibration. This is repeated three times, and the average is used to determine the VPT for each foot. VPT values of less than 15V are graded as normal and greater than 25V as severe neuropathy.[11,12,46]

Pin-prick sensation

Using a disposable pin, apply pressure just proximal to the toenail on the dorsal surface of the hallux until the skin becomes deformed. Repeat for the other foot. Patients with normal sensation will perceive the pin-prick on each foot. Inability to sense on either or both feet is abnormal.[11]

Ankle reflex

Using a percussion hammer, check the patient's ankle reflex on the Achilles tendon by holding the relaxed foot in one hand and striking the Achilles tendon with the hammer. Normal reflex will exhibit plantar flexion. This reflex becomes diminished with motor neuropathy. Providers should also test flexion and extension of the big toe and ankle.[47,48]

TRAUMA

There are multiple ways trauma to the foot can occur including, but not limited to, bony deformities, joint stiffness, and ill-fitting footwear. Any one or combination of these makes the foot susceptible to mechanical or pressure injuries and infection. Loss of peripheral sensation also makes the foot at risk for chemical and temperature traumas. Protecting the diabetic foot from these assaults is essential in the prevention of ulcer formation and/or worsening. **Table 3** provides the key elements of the complete diabetic foot examination, including the assessment for foot deformities and infections, for review.

Foot Deformity

Abnormal pressure of bony deformities can result in the formation of calluses and/or lead to ulceration. Elevated pressure on the plantar foot is another major risk factor for the development of ulcers[12,49] Structural foot deformities are very frequently concomitant with reduced joint mobility. Limited joint mobility secondary to nonenzymatic glycosylation of periarticular soft tissues combined with neuropathy can result in intrinsic muscle atrophy. With the intrinsic muscles weakened and unopposed the extrinsic muscles strength can lead to the subsequent hammering of the digits.[14] Additionally, the metatarsal heads can become more prominent and closer to the skin's surface.[50–53] Common examples of foot deformities can be seen in **Fig. 2**.

Joint Stiffness

Normal foot function relies on the ability of the hallux (great toe) to dorsiflex. Limited joint mobility can be caused by the increased thickening of both the Achilles tendon and the plantar fascia. When the range of motion of this first metatarsophalangeal joint is decreased (limitus) or immobilized (rigidus), the gait may be altered leading to increased pressure on the plantar surface of the big toe and consequently may result in ulcer formation.[49,54–56]

Ill-Fitting Footwear

A study of 440 veterans with diabetes revealed that patients with diabetic foot wounds were 5 times more likely to be wearing shoes at least one full size incorrect for their foot structure.

Shoes that are ill-fitting or no longer fit properly because of foot deformities may increase plantar pressure and friction to the skin as they rub against the bony prominences and toes causing blisters and ulcers in areas that have decreased sensation secondary to sensory neuropathy.[57–59] These sores, if not treated promptly and effectively, can develop into severe infections requiring surgery such as osteomyelitis.[60]

RISK STRATIFICATION: IDENTIFYING THE AT RISK FOOT

Following a comprehensive assessment, risk stratification helps guide health care providers and patients in determining how often the patient should be screened, as well as any necessary interventions. There are multiple organizational recommendations

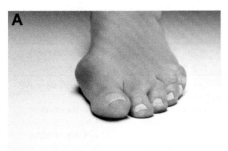 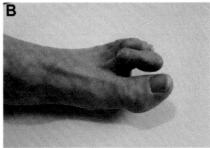

Fig. 2. Common foot deformities that increase the risk of foot ulceration. (*A*) Hallux vargus "Bunion" (*B*) Hammer toe. (Artwork [*A*] from Vasara. *Royalty-Free Stock Photo ID 714949441*. Accessed January 30, 2021. https://www.shutterstock.com/photos; Artwork [*B*] from paulaah293. *Royalty-Free Stock Photo ID:1340489969*. Accessed January 30, 2021. https://www.shutterstock.com/photos.)

for doing this but organizations consistently agree that all patients with diabetes should have a comprehensive foot examination at least one time per year.[12] **Table 6** provides a comparison of the commonly used guidelines provided by the International Working Group on the Diabetic Foot and American Diabetes Association. Both conclude that patients who fall into categories 2 and 3 should be referred to a podiatrist/foot care specialist for further evaluation and possibly diabetic footwear. Additionally, any patient who presents with an open wound or ulcer, signs of active Charcot deformity or vascular compromise should be referred to the appropriate specialist.[16,61]

ADDITIONAL INTERVENTIONS AND RECOMMENDATIONS

Diabetes is a complex and multifactorial disease. When creating a care plan, providers and patients can work to identify factors that contribute to the complications of diabetes and implement interventions to prevent them or slow their progression. Addressing these factors and incorporating clinical interventions known to reduce the risk for ulcer formation require the teamwork of both the provider(s) and patient. As previously discussed, all patients with diabetes should have a comprehensive foot examination, minimally one time per year, to evaluate for the predisposing factors for ulcer development. In addition, other modifiable known risk factors, including glycemic control, exercise, smoking, and psychological distress should be reviewed and addressed. A comprehensive approach is required to improve outcomes and decrease the risk PAD and neuropathy.

Optimizing Glycemic Control

Additional measures for ulcer and amputation prevention start with improving glycemic control. When considering risk for the development of neuropathy, higher hemoglobin A1C (HA1C) was the most significant risk factor.[62] A meta-analysis regarding

Table 6
Diabetic foot risk classification comparison and recommended frequency of examinations

Modified American Diabetes Association	• No LOPS • No PAD	• ± LOPS • ± foot deformity	• + PAD • ± LOPS • + Diminished pedal pulses • + swelling or edema	• + Chronic venous insufficiency & • + Hx of ulcer &/or • + Hx of LEA
Frequency	• Annually	• Every 4–6 mo	• Every 2–3 mo	• Every 1–2 mo
Category	**0: Very Low**	**1: Low**	**2: Moderate**	**3: High**
International Working Group on the Diabetic Foot	• No LOPS • No PAD	• + LOPS Or • + PAD	• + LOPS &+ PAD O • + LOPS & foot deformity or • + PAD & foot deformity	• +LOPS or + PAD & • + Hx of ulcer &/or • + Hx of LEA &/or • ESRD
Frequency	• Annually	• Every 6–12 mo	• Every 3–6 mo	• Every 1–3 mo

Abbreviations: ESRD, end stage renal disease; LOPS, loss of protective sensation; PAD, peripheral artery disease.
Data from Refs.[11,12,16,61]

the glycemic control and DFU outcomes suggested that persistent hyperglycemia (HA1C levels ≥8% and fasting glucose levels ≥126 mg/dL) increased the likelihood of lower extremity amputations in patients with DFU.[15] Optimizing glucose control can both delay the development of neuropathy in type 1 diabetes and slow the progression of neuropathy for patients living with type 2 diabetes. Better glycemic control is not only a factor in neuropathy but all microvascular complications.[34,63]

The risk of amputation increases in the presence of microvascular disease and is increased 22.7-fold when the patient also has peripheral arterial disease.[64] The United Kingdom Prospective Diabetes Study demonstrated a 25% reduction in microvascular complications with a 1% mean reduction in HA1C.[65]

It is recommended by the Joslin Diabetes Center that patients with diabetes set a goal for fasting blood sugar between 70 and 130 mg/dL, a 2 hour postprandial blood sugar less than 180 mg/dL, and a bedtime blood sugar between 90 and 150 mg/dL.[66] The American Diabetes Association recommends obtaining HA1C levels at minimum two times per year in patients with diabetes whose glycemic control is stable and every 3 months in patients who are not meeting glycemic goals.[67] Studies have demonstrated that frequent and consistent HA1C testing is associated with decreased complications and amputation rates.[68]

Exercise

Exercise has been a mainstay in diabetes management because of its ability to improve glucose control in diabetes. This exercise benefit can come from aerobic exercise, resistance training, or a combination of the two.[69] However, the greatest improvements in A1C are associated with higher levels of intense exercise.[70] For most patients, the ADA recommends moderate to vigorous intensity exercise three times per week for a minimum of 150 total minutes. It is also recommended to spread the activity over the course of the week, aiming to avoid more than two consecutive days without activity.[71] In addition to vigorous activity, activities such as yoga and tai chi patients may help patients maintain and improve range of motion strength and balance.[72] Another promising study on the positive effects of exercise came from the University of Utah which demonstrated nerve fiber regeneration in patients with type 2 diabetes who engaged in a regular exercise program.[31]

Smoking Cessation

Diabetics who smoke, or are exposed to second-hand smoke, have an increased risk of peripheral arterial disease, premature death, microvascular complications such as neuropathy and worse glycemic control when compared with those who do not.[73–75] As a result, smoking also increases the risk of diabetic foot amputations and can lead to vascular changes such as impaired vasodilation and increased vasoconstriction. The combination of these can lead to tissue hypoxia and interfere with the healing process.[74,76] Smoking is the most significant modifiable risk factor in the development of peripheral arterial diseases. Cessation of smoking has been shown to decrease the risk of developing intermittent claudication associated with PAD and, ultimately, decrease the subsequent risk of amputation.[2,77]

Psychological Well-Being

Multiple psychosocial factors, such as social, behavioral, and emotional factors, affect the lives of patients living with diabetes and directly affect their ability to achieve medical goals. Living with diabetes requires continued attention to medication, glucose monitoring, food, and exercise routines. The increased demands of living with diabetes and worry of disease progression may lead patients to experience significant

Table 7
Patients with diabetes foot care discussion points

Foot Examination	• Annual in clinic foot examination, or more frequent if applicable • Daily at home foot check for calluses, sores, peeling, blisters, swelling and skin health: infection, cracks; can use mirror if needed • Promptly report changes and lesions
Skin care	• Wash and thoroughly dry feet & between the toes every day with warm water • Check water temperatures with hand first to avoid thermal injury • Apply moisturizer/emollient daily to the top and bottom of the feet but avoid between the toes
Nail care	• Avoid using over-the-counter chemical products or sharp objects for the treatment of corns and calluses to avoid chemical injuries • Avoid cutting toenails too short; cut nails straight across • Reports signs of toenail infection like thickening or discoloration
Trauma protection	• Wear socks and change them daily • Wear footwear inside and outdoors • Wear well-fitting shoes ○ Breathable material, supportive, not too tight or loose, cushioned, without seams or objects that can cause friction • Check inside shoes for objects that could cause injury or friction before putting them on each time • Avoid applying heating pads on the feet or placing near heaters

Data from Refs.[12,61,80]

negative emotions and what is referred to as diabetic distress (DD). It has been reported that 18% to 45% of patients experience DD. DD can prevent patients from participating in their diabetic management and has been links to increased glucose levels and poor dietary and exercise choices. Patients identified with DD should be referred to team members, such as diabetic educators or behavioral health, to help address the areas of diabetes care most impacting the patient.[78,79]

Proper Home Foot Care

As it has been discussed previously, proper diabetic foot care is a crucial aspect in diabetic treatment because of the role they place in detecting foot problems early and preventing ulcer development or other complications. Educating patients on the importance of the foot examination includes discussing the implications of foot deformities, neuropathy, and peripheral arterial disease. In addition, patients should be informed on proper foot care, including wearing appropriate footwear, foot protective behaviors, daily foot examinations, nail, and skin care.[12,34,61,80] See **Table 7** for a list of suggestive discussion points.

SUMMARY

Patients with DM are more prone to both microvascular and macrovascular chronic complications, including neuropathy. Neuropathy can lead to a loss of sensation and bony deformations that increase the risk of ulcer formation. Additionally, patients with poorly controlled diabetes and neuropathy are at increased risk for peripheral arterial disease. PAD results in decreased blood flow and subsequently the development of lower extremity ischemia. Neuropathy, vascular disease and trauma secondary to bony deformities increase the risk of foot ulceration and possible amputation.

Regular comprehensive foot examinations allow health care providers to classify and recognize the at-risk foot and recommend appropriate early intervention to prevent complication development. This, combined with efforts to improve modifiable risk factors like glycemic control, exercise, smoking cessation, and home foot care help protect patients from developing foot ulcers, subsequent infections, amputations, and even early death.

CLINICS CARE POINTS

- Diabetes is a complex chronic disease that can lead to multiple complications including diabetic ulcers and subsequent lower extremity amputations.
- Diabetic ulcer formation occurs secondary to vascular, neuropathic, and biomechanical changes and foot deformities.
- Prevention of diabetic foot complications includes identifying the at-risk foot with comprehensive, regular foot examinations in the clinic and at home and referring for appropriate care.
- Screening for loss of protective sensation is most commonly detected using the nylon Semmes-Weinstein monofilament test and can be performed with same sensitivity at 4 points as 10.
- Assessment for peripheral arterial disease by measuring ABIs is another helpful screening test, but may be falsely elevated and require additional testing.
- Optimizing glycemic control, regular exercise, smoking cessation, and at-home foot examinations can help reduce foot ulceration.

DISCLOSURE

The author has nothing to disclose.

REFERENCES

1. Boulton AJM, Whitehouse RW. The Diabetic Foot. In: Feingold KR, Anawalt B, Boyce A, et al., eds Endotext. MDText.com, Inc.; 2000. Available at: http://www.ncbi.nlm.nih.gov/books/NBK409609/. Accessed January 30, 2021.
2. Setacci C, Benevento D, De Donato G, et al. Focusing on Diabetic Ulcers. Transl Med Unisa 2020;21:7–9.
3. Armstrong DG, Boulton AJM, Bus SA. Diabetic Foot Ulcers and Their Recurrence. N Engl J Med 2017;376(24):2367–75.
4. Lazzarini PA, Pacella RE, Armstrong DG, et al. Diabetes-related lower-extremity complications are a leading cause of the global burden of disability. Diabet Med J Br Diabet Assoc 2018. https://doi.org/10.1111/dme.13680.
5. Hicks CW, Selvarajah S, Mathioudakis N, et al. Burden of Infected Diabetic Foot Ulcers on Hospital Admissions and Costs. Ann Vasc Surg 2016;33:149–58.
6. National Diabetes Statistics Report, 2020 | CDC. Published September 28, 2020. Available at: https://www.cdc.gov/diabetes/data/statistics-report/index.html. Accessed January 30, 2021.
7. Bosiers M, Schneider P. Critical limb ischemia. 1st edition. Boca Raton: CRC Press; 2019.
8. Wukich DK, Raspovic KM, Suder NC. Patients With Diabetic Foot Disease Fear Major Lower-Extremity Amputation More Than Death. Foot Ankle Spec 2018;11(1):17–21.

9. Pendsey SP. Understanding diabetic foot. Int J Diabetes Dev Ctries 2010; 30(2):75–9.

10. Thorud JC, Plemmons B, Buckley CJ, et al. Mortality After Nontraumatic Major Amputation Among Patients With Diabetes and Peripheral Vascular Disease: A Systematic Review. J Foot Ankle Surg 2016;55(3):591–9.

11. Boulton AJM, Armstrong DG, Albert SF, et al. Comprehensive Foot Examination and Risk Assessment A report of the Task Force of the Foot Care Interest Group of the American Diabetes Association, with endorsement by the American Association of Clinical Endocrinologists. Diabetes Care 2008;31(8):1679–85.

12. Singh N, Armstrong DG, Lipsky BA. Preventing Foot Ulcers in Patients With Diabetes. JAMA 2005;293(2):217–28.

13. Dua A, Lee CJ. Epidemiology of Peripheral Arterial Disease and Critical Limb Ischemia. Tech Vasc Interv Radiol 2016;19(2):91–5.

14. Wu S, Armstrong DG, Lavery LA, et al. Clinical examination of the diabetic foot and the identification of the at-risk patient. In: Veves A, Giurini JM, Logerfo FW, editors. The diabetic foot. Contemporary diabetes. Totowa: Humana Press; 2006. p. 201–26. https://doi.org/10.1007/978-1-59745-075-1_11.

15. Lane KL, Abusamaan MS, Voss BF, et al. Glycemic control and diabetic foot ulcer outcomes: A systematic review and meta-analysis of observational studies. J Diabetes Complications 2020;34(10):107638.

16. Boulton AJM, Armstrong DG, Kirsner RS, et al. Diagnosis and management of diabetic foot complications. American Diabetes Association; 2018. Available at: http://www.ncbi.nlm.nih.gov/books/NBK538977/. Accessed January 30, 2021.

17. Sayiner ZA, Can FI, Akarsu E. Patients' clinical charecteristics and predictors for diabetic foot amputation. Prim Care Diabetes 2019;13(3):247–51.

18. Crawford F, Cezard G, Chappell FM, et al. A systematic review and individual patient data meta-analysis of prognostic factors for foot ulceration in people with diabetes: the international research collaboration for the prediction of diabetic foot ulcerations (PODUS). Health Technol Assess Winch Engl 2015;19(57):1–210.

19. Aaron Barnes J, Eid Mark A, Creager Mark A, et al. Epidemiology and Risk of Amputation in Patients With Diabetes Mellitus and Peripheral Artery Disease. Arterioscler Thromb Vasc Biol 2020;40(8):1808–17.

20. Lim JZM, Ng NSL, Thomas C. Prevention and treatment of diabetic foot ulcers. J R Soc Med 2017;110(3):104–9.

21. Musuuza J, Sutherland BL, Kurter S, et al. A systematic review of multidisciplinary teams to reduce major amputations for patients with diabetic foot ulcers. J Vasc Surg 2020;71(4):1433–46.e3.

22. Yang S-L, Zhu L-Y, Han R, et al. Pathophysiology of peripheral arterial disease in diabetes mellitus. J Diabetes 2017;9(2):133–40.

23. Hinchliffe RJ, Forsythe RO, Apelqvist J, et al. Guidelines on diagnosis, prognosis, and management of peripheral artery disease in patients with foot ulcers and diabetes (IWGDF 2019 update). Diabetes Metab Res Rev 2020;36(Suppl 1):e3276.

24. Firnhaber JM, Powell CS. Lower Extremity Peripheral Artery Disease: Diagnosis and Treatment. Am Fam Physician 2019;99(6):362–9.

25. Ibrahim A. IDF Clinical Practice Recommendation on the Diabetic Foot: A guide for healthcare professionals. Diabetes Res Clin Pract 2017;127:285–7.

26. Boyko EJ. How to use clinical signs and symptoms to estimate the probability of limb ischaemia in patients with a diabetic foot ulcer. Diabetes Metab Res Rev 2020;36(Suppl 1):e3241.

27. Suominen V, Uurto I, Saarinen J, et al. PAD as a risk factor for mortality among patients with elevated ABI–a clinical study. Eur J Vasc Endovasc Surg 2010; 39(3):316–22.

28. Xu null D, Li null J, Zou null L, et al. Sensitivity and specificity of the ankle–brachial index to diagnose peripheral artery disease: a structured review. Vasc Med Lond Engl 2010;15(5):361–9.

29. Donohue CM, Adler JV, Bolton LL. Peripheral arterial disease screening and diagnostic practice: A scoping review. Int Wound J 2020;17(1):32–44.

30. Hicks CW, Selvin E. Epidemiology of Peripheral Neuropathy and Lower Extremity Disease in Diabetes. Curr Diab Rep 2019;19(10):86.

31. Pop-Busui R, Boulton AJM, Feldman EL, et al. Diabetic Neuropathy: A Position Statement by the American Diabetes Association. Diabetes Care 2017;40(1): 136–54.

32. Dardari D. An overview of Charcot's neuroarthropathy. J Clin Transl Endocrinol 2020;22:100239.

33. Trieb K. The Charcot foot: pathophysiology, diagnosis and classification. Bone Joint J 2016;98-B(9):1155–9.

34. Association AD. Microvascular Complications and Foot Care: Standards of Medical Care in Diabetes—2018. Diabetes Care 2018;41(Supplement 1):S105–18.

35. Mark Jacobs A. A Closer Look At Motor Neuropathy In Patients With Diabetes. Podiatry Today 2008;21(9):44–52.

36. Andersen H. Motor neuropathy. Handb Clin Neurol 2014;126:81–95.

37. Akkuş G, Evran M, Güngör D, et al. Tinea pedis and onychomycosis frequency in diabetes mellitus patients and diabetic foot ulcers: A cross sectional – observational study | Akkuş | Pakistan Journal of Medical Sciences Old Website. Available at: http://www.pjms.com.pk/index.php/pjms/article/view/10027. Accessed January 30, 2021.

38. Feng Y, Schlösser FJ, Sumpio BE. The Semmes Weinstein monofilament examination is a significant predictor of the risk of foot ulceration and amputation in patients with diabetes mellitus. J Vasc Surg 2011;53(1):220–6.e1-5.

39. Mayfield JA, Sugarman JR. The use of the Semmes-Weinstein monofilament and other threshold tests for preventing foot ulceration and amputation in persons with diabetes. J Fam Pract 2000;49(11 Suppl):S17–29.

40. Nather A, Keng Lin W, Aziz Z, et al. Assessment of sensory neuropathy in patients with diabetic foot problems. Diabet Foot Ankle 2011;2. https://doi.org/10.3402/dfa.v2i0.6367.

41. Dros J, Wewerinke A, Bindels PJ, et al. Accuracy of monofilament testing to diagnose peripheral neuropathy: a systematic review. Ann Fam Med 2009;7(6):555–8.

42. Feng Y, Schlösser FJ, Sumpio BE. The Semmes Weinstein monofilament examination as a screening tool for diabetic peripheral neuropathy. J Vasc Surg 2009;50(3):675–82, 682.e1.

43. Lanting SM, Spink MJ, Tehan PE, et al. Non-invasive assessment of vibration perception and protective sensation in people with diabetes mellitus: inter- and intra-rater reliability. J Foot Ankle Res 2020;13(1):3.

44. Zhang Q, Yi N, Liu S, et al. Easier operation and similar power of 10 g monofilament test for screening diabetic peripheral neuropathy. J Int Med Res 2018;46(8): 3278–84.

45. Lavery LA, Lavery DE, Lavery DC, et al. Accuracy and durability of Semmes–Weinstein monofilaments: What is the useful service life? Diabetes Res Clin Pract 2012;97(3):399–404.

46. Medakkel A, Sheela P. Vibration Perception Threshold Values and Clinical Symptoms of Diabetic Peripheral Neuropathy. J Clin Diagn Res 2018;12:YC05–8.
47. Malik MM, Jindal S, Bansal S, et al. Relevance of ankle reflex as a screening test for diabetic peripheral neuropathy. Indian J Endocrinol Metab 2013;17(Suppl1):S340–1.
48. Francia P, Seghieri G, Gulisano M, et al. The role of joint mobility in evaluating and monitoring the risk of diabetic foot ulcer. Diabetes Res Clin Pract 2015;108(3):398–404.
49. Tang UH, Zügner R, Lisovskaja V, et al. Foot deformities, function in the lower extremities, and plantar pressure in patients with diabetes at high risk to develop foot ulcers. Diabet Foot Ankle 2015;6:27593.
50. Wrobel JS, Najafi B. Diabetic foot biomechanics and gait dysfunction. J Diabetes Sci Technol 2010;4(4):833–45.
51. DiPreta JA. Metatarsalgia, lesser toe deformities, and associated disorders of the forefoot. Med Clin North Am 2014;98(2):233–51.
52. Kwon O, Tuttle L, Johnson J, et al. Muscle imbalance and reduced ankle joint motion in people with hammer toe deformity. Clin Biomech (Bristol Avon) 2009;24(8):670–5.
53. Hagedorn TJ, Dufour AB, Riskowski JL, et al. Foot disorders, foot posture, and foot function: the Framingham foot study. PLoS One 2013;8(9):e74364.
54. Park CH, Chang MC. Forefoot disorders and conservative treatment. Yeungnam Univ J Med 2019;36(2):92–8.
55. Allan J, Munro W, Figgins E. Foot deformities within the diabetic foot and their influence on biomechanics: A review of the literature. Prosthet Orthot Int 2016;40(2):182–92.
56. Yu G, Fan Y, Fan Y, et al. The Role of Footwear in the Pathogenesis of Hallux Valgus: A Proof-of-Concept Finite Element Analysis in Recent Humans and Homo naledi. Front Bioeng Biotechnol 2020;8. https://doi.org/10.3389/fbioe.2020.00648.
57. Reiber GE, Vileikyte L, Boyko EJ, et al. Causal pathways for incident lower-extremity ulcers in patients with diabetes from two settings. Diabetes Care 1999;22(1):157–62.
58. Nixon BP, Armstrong DG, Wendell C, et al. Do US veterans wear appropriately sized shoes?: the Veterans Affairs shoe size selection study. J Am Podiatr Med Assoc 2006;96(4):290–2.
59. Branthwaite H, Chockalingam N, Greenhalgh A. The effect of shoe toe box shape and volume on forefoot interdigital and plantar pressures in healthy females. J Foot Ankle Res 2013;6(1):28.
60. Pitocco D, Spanu T, Di Leo M, et al. Diabetic foot infections: a comprehensive overview. Eur Rev Med Pharmacol Sci 2019;23(2 Suppl):26–37.
61. Bus SA, Lavery LA, Monteiro-Soares M, et al. Guidelines on the prevention of foot ulcers in persons with diabetes (IWGDF 2019 update). Diabetes Metab Res Rev 2020;36(Suppl 1):e3269.
62. Braffett BH, Gubitosi-Klug RA, Albers JW, et al. Risk Factors for Diabetic Peripheral Neuropathy and Cardiovascular Autonomic Neuropathy in the Diabetes Control and Complications Trial/Epidemiology of Diabetes Interventions and Complications (DCCT/EDIC) Study. Diabetes 2020;69(5):1000–10.
63. Effect of intensive diabetes treatment on nerve conduction in the diabetes control and complications trial. Ann Neurol 1995;38(6):869–80.

64. Beckman Joshua A, Duncan Meredith S, Damrauer Scott M, et al. Microvascular Disease, Peripheral Artery Disease, and Amputation. Circulation 2019;140(6): 449–58.
65. Effect of intensive blood-glucose control with metformin on complications in overweight patients with type 2 diabetes (UKPDS 34). UK Prospective Diabetes Study (UKPDS) Group. Lancet 1998;352(9131):854–65.
66. Goals for Glucose Control. Joslin Diabetes Center. Available at: https://www.joslin. org/patient-care/diabetes-education/diabetes-learning-center/goals-glucose-control. Accessed January 30, 2021.
67. Parcero AF, Yaeger T, Bienkowski RS. Frequency of Monitoring Hemoglobin A1C and Achieving Diabetes Control. J Prim Care Community Health 2011;2(3):205–8.
68. Suckow BD, Newhall KA, Bekelis K, et al. Hemoglobin A1c Testing and Amputation Rates in Black, Hispanic, and White Medicare Patients. Ann Vasc Surg 2016; 36:208–17.
69. Umpierre D, Ribeiro PAB, Kramer CK, et al. Physical activity advice only or structured exercise training and association with HbA1c levels in type 2 diabetes: a systematic review and meta-analysis. JAMA 2011;305(17):1790–9.
70. Boulé NG, Kenny GP, Haddad E, et al. Meta-analysis of the effect of structured exercise training on cardiorespiratory fitness in Type 2 diabetes mellitus. Diabetologia 2003;46(8):1071–81.
71. Association AD. 5. Lifestyle Management: Standards of Medical Care in Diabetes—2019. Diabetes Care 2019;42(Supplement 1):S46–60.
72. Kirwan JP, Sacks J, Nieuwoudt S. The essential role of exercise in the management of type 2 diabetes. Cleve Clin J Med 2017;84(7 Suppl 1):S15–21.
73. Willigendael EM, Teijink JAW, Bartelink M-L, et al. Influence of smoking on incidence and prevalence of peripheral arterial disease. J Vasc Surg 2004;40(6): 1158–65.
74. Xia N, Morteza A, Yang F, et al. Review of the role of cigarette smoking in diabetic foot. J Diabetes Investig 2019;10(2):202–15.
75. Clair C, Cohen MJ, Eichler F, et al. The Effect of Cigarette Smoking on Diabetic Peripheral Neuropathy: A Systematic Review and Meta-Analysis. J Gen Intern Med 2015;30(8):1193–203.
76. Liu M, Zhang W, Yan Z, et al. Smoking increases the risk of diabetic foot amputation: A meta-analysis. Exp Ther Med 2018;15(2):1680–5.
77. Bevan Graham H, White Solaru Khendi T. Evidence-Based Medical Management of Peripheral Artery Disease. Arterioscler Thromb Vasc Biol 2020;40(3):541–53.
78. Aikens JE. Prospective associations between emotional distress and poor outcomes in type 2 diabetes. Diabetes Care 2012;35(12):2472–8.
79. Snoek FJ, Bremmer MA, Hermanns N. Constructs of depression and distress in diabetes: time for an appraisal. Lancet Diabetes Endocrinol 2015;3(6):450–60.
80. Diabetes and You: Healthy Feet Matter! Diabetes and Your Feet. 2014. Available at: https://www.cdc.gov/diabetes/ndep/pdfs/toolkits/working-together/151-health-feet-matter.pdf. Accessed January 30, 2021.

Update on Cardiovascular Disease Prevention

Jonathan Kilstrom, MPAS, PA-C, NRP[a],*, Anne Wildermuth, MMS, PA-C, EM CAQ, RD[b]

KEYWORDS

- Cardiovascular disease • Atherosclerotic cardiovascular disease • Prevention
- Diabetes • Hypertension • Aspirin • Fish oil • CT calcium score

KEY POINTS

- In the United States, cardiovascular disease (CVD) is the leading cause of death for men, women, and nearly every racial and ethnic group.
- The decision to begin low-dose aspirin for the primary prevention of CVD should be done on a case-by-case basis following the established USPSTF guidelines.
- Focusing on lifestyle modifications, smoking cessation, and optimizing control of diseases that increase CVD risk is critical for prevention.
- Calculating the 10-year atherosclerotic CVD risk is critical to optimize and individualize patient management and prevention strategies.

INTRODUCTION

In the United States, cardiovascular disease (CVD) is the leading cause of death for men, women, and nearly every racial and ethnic group, accounting for approximately 655,000 deaths per year[1] (Table 1). Coronary artery disease is the most common type of CVD, affecting about 18.2 million adults and was responsible for 365,914 deaths in 2017.[1] Approximately, 805,000 Americans have a myocardial infarction each year, of which, approximately, 605,000 are a first-time event.[1]

Hypertension (HTN), hyperlipidemia, and tobacco abuse are key risk factors for CVD.[1] Other modifiable risk factors for CVD include history of diabetes, obesity, poor diet, physical inactivity, and excessive alcohol use.[1]

Costs of health care services, medications, and loss of productivity due to death secondary to CVD reached a staggering $219 billion in the United States from 2014

Neither author has any commercial or financial conflicts of interest.
[a] Yale University School of Medicine, Physician Assistant Online Program, PO Box 208004, New Haven, CT 06520-8004, USA; [b] Department of Physician Assistant Studies, The George Washington University School of Medicine and Health Sciences, 2300 Eye Street Northwest, Suite 226, Washington, DC 20052, USA
* Corresponding author.
E-mail address: jonathan.kilstrom@yale.edu

Table 1
Percentages of all deaths caused by cardiovascular disease in 2015[1]

Race of Ethic Group	% of Deaths	Men, %	Women, %
American Indian or Alaska Native	18.3	19.4	17.0
Asian American or Pacific Islander	21.4	22.9	19.9
Black (Non-Hispanic)	23.5	23.9	23.1
White (Non-Hispanic)	23.7	24.9	22.5
Hispanic	20.3	20.6	19.9
All	23.4	24.4	22.3

Table adapted from CDC, open source.

to 2015.[1] The exorbitant costs secondary to CVD in addition to the high number of Americans affected highlights the importance of disease prevention.

DISCUSSION
Goals

In 2019, the American Heart Association (AHA) and American College of Cardiology (ACC) published comprehensive guidelines on primary prevention of CVD.[2] Included in these guidelines are several goals related to lifestyle modification and diet. Although reaching these goals as quickly as is reasonable is important for CVD prevention, long-term compliance is of particular importance. Because some of these lifestyle and diet changes will be considerable for some patients, working with the patient to set reachable goals is important for long-term compliance. A team-based approach to managing care is essential, and social determinants of health relevant to individual patients should be considered when recommending prevention strategies.[2]

Diet

A well-balanced diet of fruits and vegetables, lean meat and fish, nuts, and whole grains is optimal for reducing CVD risk. In addition to rising rates of obesity in the U.S., observational studies indicate a correlation between CVD mortality and consumption of sugar, low-calorie sweeteners, high-carbohydrate diets, low-carbohydrate diets, refined grains, trans fat, saturated fat, sodium, red meat, and processed red meat.[2] As such, these foods should be limited and avoided when possible.[2] Both a plant-based diet and the Mediterranean diet are associated with lower all-cause mortality and lower CVD risk and should be encouraged.[2] The Mediterranean diet lacks a specific definition but is generally high in fruits, vegetables, whole grains, nuts, seeds, and olive oil.[3] As the Mediterranean diet is primarily plant based, lean white meat, fish, and small amounts of dairy may be included; red meat is limited or absent.[3] The plant-based diet, whereby animal protein is replaced with vegetable protein, is associated with a considerable reduction in CVD mortality in two large clinical trials, PREDIMED and the Adventist Health Study-2.[2] Regardless of the diet selected, saturated fats and trans fats should be avoided; a reduction in cholesterol intake is also beneficial.[2] Patients should be encouraged to limit sodium consumption to less than 1500 mg (1.5 g) daily.[2]

Alcohol

Per the 2020–2025 Dietary Guidelines for Americans (DGA), adult men should drink less than 2 drinks daily and adult women should drink less than 1 drink daily; abstinence from alcohol is also reasonable.[4] Alcohol consumption is associated with

HTN, an important risk factor for CVD, and consuming alcohol in moderation per the DGA, if at all, should be encouraged.[2]

Exercise

Completion of 150 minutes of moderate-intensity exercise or 75 minutes of high-intensity exercise each week is recommended to reduce risk of CVD; a combination of moderate- and high-intensity exercise is acceptable.[2] Moderate-intensity activity includes, but is not limited to, brisk walking, bicycle riding (6–9 miles per hour), and recreational swimming; high-intensity activity encompasses running, swimming laps, and singles tennis among others.[2] At health care maintenance visits, patients should be encouraged to maintain as active of a lifestyle as possible. Even if the recommended exercise goals can be met, completion of any physical activity and avoidance of a sedentary lifestyle likely is beneficial in reducing risk of CVD.[2] Prescribing exercise that aligns with the aforementioned Centers for Disease Control guidelines including type, duration, intensity, and frequency may improve compliance and is recommended.[2]

Smoking

Smoking, smokeless tobacco, and secondhand smoke increase all-cause mortality and risk of CVD; it is the leading preventable cause of death in the U.S.[2] Adults who use tobacco should be advised and supported with cessation; individuals should also avoid secondhand smoke.[2] A combination of behavioral and pharmacologic therapy, in addition to strict avoidance of tobacco, is recommended to increase success of cessation. It is critical that providers ask about smoking, the use of any tobacco product, and even limited use of any tobacco product to determine smoking status at every visit, as asking "Are you a smoker?" may not elicit the desired information.[2] Even very limited tobacco use is associated with an increased risk of CVD, so strict avoidance is important.[2] It may be helpful and increase cessation success to have a dedicated tobacco cessation team or expert involved in managing patient care.

DISEASE AFFECTING CARDIOVASCULAR RISK

Overweight and obesity, diabetes mellitus, high serum cholesterol, and HTN all increase risk for CVD; effectively managing these diseases helps with CVD prevention and risk reduction.[2]

In adults with overweight or obesity, weight loss is recommended until a normal body mass index (BMI) of less than 25 is achieved; BMI should be calculated at least annually.[2] All adults with overweight or obesity should be referred to a comprehensive lifestyle program, either in person or virtually, for more than 6 months to assist patients in following a low-calorie diet and achieving exercise goals.[2] A reasonable calorie goal for most adults with overweight or obesity is 1200 to 1500 kcal/d for women and 1500 to 1800 kcal/d for men.[2]

Type 2 diabetes mellitus (T2DM) or a hemoglobin A1C more than 6.5%, is a disease characterized by insulin resistance; it is a significant risk factor for atherosclerotic CVD (ASCVD). T2DM is heavily associated with weight, diet, and physical activity.[2] Improved glycemic control significantly reduces ASCVD risk, and it is important to counsel patients to follow a heart healthy diet, exercise, and lose weight if needed as previously outlined.[2] In addition to these lifestyle modifications, metformin should be initiated as first-line therapy to improve glycemic control.[2] Some patients with T2DM may require an additional agent to achieve glycemic control; sodium glucose cotransporter 2 inhibitors and glucagon-like peptide-1 receptor agonists may help reduce ASCVD risk and lower serum glucose.[2]

High serum cholesterol is a known risk factor for ASCVD, and it is important to assess 10-year estimated cardiac risk in adults aged 40 to 75 years to guide management.[2] A heart healthy diet should be encouraged to all patients. In young adults aged 20 to 39 years, drug therapy is considered when low-density lipoprotein (LDL) level is > 160 mg/dL (moderate) and typically prescribed when LDL is > 190 mg/dL (high).[2,5] Patients aged 75 years and older should undergo shared decision-making with the clinician on the benefits and risks of pharmacologic therapy.[2,5] Risk stratification ideally occurs using the Pooled Cohort Equation (PCE) in non-Hispanic whites and blacks; other risk assessment tools like the Framingham CVD Risk Score or Reynolds Score may be preferred in other racial or ethnic groups because PCE can overestimate or underestimate risk in these patients.[2] In the PCE, risk stratification is characterized as low (<5%), borderline (5% to <7.5%), intermediate (≥7.5% to <20%), or high (≥20%) 10-year risk.[2,5] Initial pharmacologic treatment of high serum cholesterol is with a statin drug, which are 3-hydroxy-3-methylglutaryl coenzyme A reductase inhibitors. Statins are prescribed in different strengths depending on risk; the higher the intensity of the statin, the greater the LDL reduction (**Table 2**).[2,5] Additionally, there are several factors that may additionally increase risk, and these enhancers may warrant additional consideration of initiating statin therapy or intensifying statin therapy. These risk enhancers include family history of ASCVD at a young age, persistently elevated LDL levels greater than 160 mg/dL, chronic kidney disease, metabolic syndrome, premature menopause, preeclampsia, inflammatory diseases, ethnicity, persistently elevated serum triglyceride levels greater than 175 mg/dL, abnormal ankle–brachial index (ABI), and other lab abnormalities of high-sensitivity C-reactive protein (hs-CRP), Lipoprotein (a), Apolipoprotein B.[2,5] Patients at intermediate risk may benefit from coronary artery calcium (CAC) measurement to assess whether a medium- or high-intensity statin is indicated if pharmacologic therapy is initiated. Certain subgroups are known to significantly benefit from statin therapy, and it should be started in these patients whenever possible (**Table 3**).[2,5]

HTN, defined as systolic blood pressure ≥ 130 mm Hg or diastolic blood pressure ≥ 80 mm Hg, is the biggest contributor to deaths from ASCVD of any modifiable risk factor. Stage I HTN is defined as a blood pressure of 130 to 139/80 to 80 mm Hg, and stage 2 HTN is defined as blood pressure greater than 140/90.[2,6] HTN is very common worldwide, and in the U.S., it occurs more frequently in blacks than in whites, Asians, and Hispanics.[2] Per the 2017 AHA and ACC released Hypertension Clinical Practice Guidelines, all adults with HTN should have nonpharmacologic therapy recommended to lower blood pressure including weight loss if needed, heart healthy diet, sodium restriction, increased dietary potassium, increased physical activity, and limited alcohol.[2,6] The Dietary Approaches to Stop Hypertension (DASH) diet is an effective diet option to reduce blood pressure within weeks and involves consuming less than 1500 mg sodium daily and focuses on consumption of fruits, vegetables,

Table 2
Intensity of commonly prescribed statins[5]

High Intensity	Medium Intensity	Low Intensity
Atorvastatin 40–80 mg	Atorvastatin 10–20 mg	Simvastatin 10 mg
Rosuvastatin 20–40 mg	Rosuvastatin 5–10 mg	
	Simvastatin 20–40 mg	

Table 3
Statin prescribing in selected risk groups[2,5]

Risk Factor	Pharmacologic Management
LDL ≥ 190 mg/dL	High-intensity statin
Diabetes mellitus and age 40–75 years	Moderate-intensity statin; perform risk assessment to determine risk/benefit of high-intensity statin
Borderline risk (5% to <7.5%)	If risk enhancers present, risk/benefit discussion about medium-intensity statin
Intermediate risk (≥7.5% to 20%)	If risk estimate and risk enhancers suggest statin treatment, initiate moderate-intensity statin to reduce LDL by 30% to 49%. If uncertain risk, consider CAC measurement. CAC of 1–99 favors statin use; CAC of ≥100 should be prescribed a statin.
High risk (≥20%)	Initiate statin to reduce LDL by ≥ 50%

whole grains, and low-fat dairy.[7] Lean meats, fish, and legumes are also a part of the DASH diet.[7] Specific comorbid diseases and blood pressure thresholds additionally benefit from pharmacologic therapy (**Table 4**).[2,6] The primary pharmacologic agents used to treat HTN, proven to reduce the risk of cardiac events, include thiazide diuretics, angiotensin-converting enzyme (ACE) inhibitors, angiotensin receptor blockers (ARBs), and calcium channel blockers (CCBs). For adults with stage 2 HTN, it may be desirable to initially prescribe two agents of different classes; ACE inhibitors and ARBs should not be concurrently prescribed.[2,6] Consideration of hypotension risk is advisable in older adults when starting two agents concurrently; caution is advised.[6] Thiazide diuretics and CCBs are the best initial agents for black patients; ACE inhibitors and ARBs are less effective in this population.[6]

CURRENT STUDIES AND TRIALS
Low-Dose Aspirin

The use of acetylsalicylic acid (aspirin) for the primary prevention of CVD is controversial and has been widely debated for decades. In addition to its antiinflammatory, analgesic, and antipyretic effects secondary to inhibition of the cyclooxygenase enzyme-2, aspirin also inhibits the COX-1 enzyme, which results in vasodilation, reduction of platelet aggregation, and reduction of thrombus formation.[8,9]

Multiple studies looking at aspirin's effect on primary prevention of CVD performed before 2000 suggested a reduction in myocardial infarction and stroke.[9] Most of these

Table 4
Indications for pharmacologic therapy in adults with hypertension and BP target[6]

Clinical Condition	BP Target
Stage 1 HTN and > 10% 10-y CVD risk	–
Stage 2 HTN	<130/80
HTN and chronic kidney disease	<130/80
HTN and T2DM	Initiate at BP > 130/80; target is < 130/80
HTN and no other risk factors	Consider target of <130/80

studies also showed an increase in adverse bleeding events and no reduction in mortality rates.[9] In 1985, the Food and Drug Administration approved aspirin to be used for secondary prevention of CVD after reviewing a meta-analysis of individually inconclusive trials, but to date, it has not approved labeling of aspirin for primary CVD prevention.[9]

Multiple contemporary trials have reevaluated aspirin's safety and efficacy for the primary prevention of CVD. A 2019 meta-analysis concluded that, "aspirin use does not reduce all-cause or cardiovascular mortality and results in an insufficient benefit-risk ratio for CVD primary prevention."[10] The analysis also concluded non-smokers, patients treated with statins, and men had the greatest risk reduction of major adverse cardiovascular events across subgroups.[10]

The 2009 update of the U.S. Preventive Services Task Force (USPSTF)[11] on aspirin use for the primary prevention of CVD recommends initiating low-dose aspirin for the primary prevention of CVD in adults aged 50 to 59 years who have a 10% or greater 10-year CVD risk[12], are not at increased risk for bleeding, have a life expectancy of at least 10 years, and are willing to take low-dose aspirin daily for at least 10 years[11] (**Table 5**).

The USPSTF is currently undergoing a routine update regarding its recommendation on the use of aspirin for primary prevention of CVD.[13] These recommendations have not yet been published.

Fish Oil

Omega-3 fatty acid supplementation has been widely studied. Although it appears that omega-3 fatty acid supplementation is beneficial for those with underlying CVD, several large study trials (Vitamin D and Omega-3 Trial [VITAL],[14] A Study of Cardiovascular Events iN Diabetes [ASCEND],[15] Japan EPA Lipid Intervention Study [JELIS][16]) have provided evidence that the use of omega-3 fatty acid supplementation in otherwise healthy and diabetic patients without underlying cardiovascular risk factors is not effective in the primary prevention of adverse cardiovascular events[17] (**Table 6**).

The 2016 European guidelines on primary prevention of CVD conclude the protective effects of omega-3 fatty acid supplementation at reducing all-cause CAD and stroke mortality is debatable.[18] The 2017 AHA guidelines have issued a "no recommendation" for initiating omega-3 fatty acid supplementation for the primary prevention of coronary heart disease (CHD) in the general population due to a lack of randomized controlled trials that have targeted exclusively the primary prevention of CHD in the general population of patients without prior CHD.[19] (Final findings of the VITAL trial had not yet been published.)

AHA guidelines do not recommend initiating omega-3 supplementation for the primary prevention of CVD mortality in patients with diabetes/prediabetes and those at high risk of CVD (class III recommendation).[19]

AHA guidelines do indicate that treatment for secondary prevention of CHD with omega-3 fatty acid supplementation is reasonable (class IIa) among patients with prevalent CHD and among patients with heart failure.[19]

CT CALCIUM SCORE TESTING

The PCE is considered a more contemporary global risk score than the Framingham Risk Score and is currently being used to estimate the 10-year ASCVD risk in the ACC/AHA cholesterol guidelines and in the 2016 USPSTF guidelines.[20]

Although the exact reasons are unclear, multiple external validation cohorts have shown that the PCE tends to overestimate actual CVD risk.[21]

Table 5
Aspirin use for the primary prevention of cardiovascular disease: clinical summary[11]

Population	Recommendation	Grade
Adults aged 50–59 y with a ≥10% 10-y CVD risk	The USPSTF recommends initiating low-dose aspirin use for the primary prevention of cardiovascular disease (CVD) in adults aged 50–59 y who have a 10% or greater 10-y CVD risk, are not at increased risk for bleeding, have a life expectancy of at least 10 y, and are willing to take low-dose aspirin daily for at least 10 y.	B
Adults aged 60–69 y with a ≥10% 10-y CVD risk	The decision to initiate low-dose aspirin use for the primary prevention of CVD in adults aged 60–69 y who have a 10% or greater 10-y CVD risk should be an individual one. Persons who are not at increased risk for bleeding, have a life expectancy of at least 10 y, and are willing to take low-dose aspirin daily for at least 10 y are more likely to benefit. Persons who place a higher value on the potential benefits than the potential harms may choose to initiate low-dose aspirin.	C
Adults aged 70 y or older	The current evidence is insufficient to assess the balance of benefits and harms of initiating aspirin use for the primary prevention of CVD.	I
Adults younger than 50 y	The current evidence is insufficient to assess the balance of benefits and harms of initiating aspirin use for the primary prevention of CVD.	I

Abbreviations: ACC/AHA, American College of Cardiology/American Heart Association; CVD, cardiovascular disease; GI, gastrointestinal.
Taken from U.S. Preventive Services Task Force, open source.

Although the Framingham Risk Score and the PCE estimate CV risk based on mean risk factor distributions across a population, the CAC score provides an individualized direct marker of atherosclerosis and has been shown to be reliable, reproducible, and predictive of adverse cardiovascular outcomes.[20,22]

For patients with uncertain quantitative risk-based assessment using the PCE or Framingham Risk Score, ACC/AHA recommend assessing CAC score, family history, hs-CRP, or ABI in order to make an informed treatment decision.[23] Recent studies have demonstrated that when compared with brachial flow-mediated dilation, ABI, carotid intima-media thickness, and hs-CRP, CAC scores remain the strongest test for reclassifying events when used with PCE.[20]

The 10-year risk for ASCVD is categorized as follows: low risk (<5%), borderline risk (5% - 7.4%), intermediate risk (7.5% - 19.9%), and high risk (≥20%).[23] The ACC/AHA recommends measuring CAC in adults aged 40 to 75 years without diabetes mellitus

Table 6
Recent trails on fatty acid supplementation and primary prevention of CVD[14-16]

Study	Supplement and Dose	Inclusion Criteria	Effect on Primary Prevention of CVD
ASCEND (2019) (Effects of n−3 Fatty Acid Supplements in Diabetes Mellitus, n.d., #)	1 g capsule daily (containing n-3 fatty acid 840 mg and -EPA 380 mg)	>40 y, diabetic, no previous CV disease	No significant difference in the risk of serious vascular events between study and placebo groups.
VITAL research group (2019) (Marine n−3 Fatty Acids and Prevention of Cardiovascular Disease and Cancer, n.d., #)	1 g capsule daily (containing n-3 fatty acid 840 mg and EPA 380 mg)	Men ≥50 y, women ≥55 y with no history of CV disease	N-3 fatty acid supplementation did not result in a lower incidence of major CV events or cancer than placebo.
JELIS Trial (2007) (Effects of eicosapentaenoic acid on major coronary events in hypercholesterolaemic patients (JELIS): a randomised open-label, blinded endpoint analysis, n.d., #)	EPA 1800 mg with statin	Japanese patients with a total cholesterol 5.6 mmol/L or greater	In patients with no history of CAD, EPA treatment reduced coronary events by 18% but was not considered significant compared with the control group ($P = .132$)

Abbreviations: CAD, coronary artery disease; CV, cardiovascular; EPA, eicosapentaenoic acid.
  Table created by author.

and with LDL-C levels ≥70 mg/dL to 189 mg/dL and who have a 10-year ASCVD risk of ≥7.5 to 19.9% with whom a current decision about statin therapy is uncertain.[5] If CAC score is 1 to 99, statin therapy is favored, especially in those ≥55 years of age.[23] Statin therapy should be initiated in any patient with a CAC score ≥100 Agatston units or ≥75 percentile, unless the clinician–patient risk discussion deems it inappropriate.[23]

A multiethnic study of atherosclerosis published in 2015 concluded that significant ASCVD risk heterogeneity exists among those eligible for statins according to the ACC/AHA guidelines.[24] The study provided strong evidence that a CAC score of 0 can downwardly reclassify risk in patients with a 10-year ASCVD score between 5% and 15% and modest evidence that a CAC score of 0 can downwardly reclassify risk in patients between 15% and 20% to a level that statin therapy would not be recommended. Patients with a 10-year ASCVD risk score greater than 20% are considered high risk regardless of the CAC score.[24]

Evaluation

Evaluation of patients for CVD is multifaceted and involves a thorough history, detailed physical examination, and diagnostic studies.

It is important for clinicians to assess the 10-year ASCVD risk, typically using the PCE; the ACC has this risk estimator easily available on the Internet.[12] Successful completion of the PCE requires the patient's age, sex, race, blood pressure, serum cholesterol (total, high-density lipoprotein, LDL), and information about diabetes, HTN, smoking, statin use, and aspirin therapy.[12] Additionally, inquiries into risk enhancers are a likely fruitful component of history taking once the 10-year ASCVD risk is established to determine optimal management.[2] Smoking status should be determined at every visit.[2]

Regarding the role of electrocardiography (ECG), the U.S. Preventative Services Task Force (USPSTF) does not advise the use of screening ECG in patients at low risk for CVD.[25] There is inconclusive evidence to make a recommendation regarding the role of screening ECG in patients at moderate or higher risk of CVD.[25] As such, it is not routinely recommended for any patient to undergo screening ECG when assessing CVD risk and optimizing prevention of CVD.[25]

The physical examination when evaluating a patient for CVD risk is aimed at assessing general health and identification and monitoring of diseases that increased CVD risk, including obesity, diabetes, high cholesterol, and diabetes. Anthropometric data including a BMI at least annually and a complete set of vital signs, specifically including an accurate blood pressure, are essential.[2,6] In order to diagnose HTN, $\geq$ 2 elevated blood pressure readings should be obtained on $\geq$ 2 occasions, with the pressures being averaged.[6] A complete physical examination, with specific attention to the skin, eyes, heart, lungs, and abdomen, and vascular and neurologic examinations should be performed.

Laboratory testing involves screening for and assessment of known CVD risk factors, including T2DM, HTN, and high serum cholesterol. In order to determine 10-year ASCVD risk, a lipid panel must be performed. The USPSTF advises screening for diabetes in adults aged 40 to 70 years who are overweight or obese.[26] In patients with known HTN, basic laboratory testing includes a complete blood count, basic metabolic profile (including fasting glucose), urinalysis, lipid panel, thyroid-stimulating hormone levels, and an ECG.[6]

APPROACH TO PATIENT EDUCATION

Patient education is critically important in preventing CVD. In order to be effective at providing education, it is important to understand the patient's health literacy level and communicate accordingly.[2] Additionally, assessing the patient's motivation for change and social and environmental barriers is of critical importance.[2] Some of the aforementioned lifestyle modifications aimed at CVD prevention will represent a significant departure from the patient's current daily habits. As such, setting small, reachable goals with frequent follow-up may improve compliance, for example, gradually building up over a period of weeks or months from 10 minutes of slow walking daily to 30 minutes of brisk walking 5 times or more per week. The use of an interdisciplinary team, including registered dietitians, smoking cessation counselors, and experts on obesity management, is advisable when at all possible.[2]

SUMMARY

The primary prevention of CVD should be approached on a case-by-case basis using evidence-based predictor tools such as the 10-year ASCVD risk score and additional diagnostic testing such as laboratory values, ABI, and CAC scores as indicated.

The decision to initiate low-dose aspirin for the primary prevention of CVD should also be approached on a case-by-case basis after assessing the patient's 10-year ASCVD risk score, comorbid conditions, risk of bleeding, and current life expectancy.

Proper patient education on CVD prevention is extremely important. All patients should be encouraged to manage a healthy weight, limit alcohol consumption, avoid tobacco products, exercise regularly, and consume a diet primarily composed of fruits, vegetables, lean meat and fish, nuts, and whole grains.

CLINICS CARE POINTS

- The decision to begin low-dose aspirin for the primary prevention of cardiovascular disease (CVD) should be done on a case-by-case basis following the established U.S. Preventative Services Task Force guidelines.

- Omega-3 fish oil supplementation in patients without underlying CVD and those with diabetes mellitus currently shows no benefit in the primary prevention of CVD.

- Using coronary artery calcium scoring with the 10-year atherosclerotic CVD risk score for certain patient populations is beneficial in guiding decision-making regarding initiation of statin therapy.

- Plant-based and Mediterranean diets lower CVD risk and are recommended; additionally, sodium should be limited to less than 1.5 g daily, and alcohol should be consumed in moderation if at all.

- BMI should be measured at least annually, and all adults who are overweight or obese should be referred to a comprehensive lifestyle program to guide weight loss efforts.

- Smoking status should be inquired about at every visit; advising and support for smoking cessation with pharmacologic and behavioral interventions is optimal.

REFERENCES

1. CDC. Heart disease facts. Cdc.gov. 2020. Available at: https://www.cdc.gov/heartdisease/facts.htm. Accessed January 13, 2021.
2. Arnett DK, Blumenthal RS, Albert MA, et al. 2019 ACC/AHA guideline on the primary prevention of cardiovascular disease: a report of the American College of Cardiology/American Heart Association Task Force on clinical practice guidelines [published correction appears in Circulation. 2019 Sep 10;140(11):e649-e650] [published correction appears in Circulation. 2020 Jan 28;141(4):e60] [published correction appears in Circulation. 2020 Apr 21;141(16):e774]. Circulation 2019; 140(11):e596–646.
3. Mayo Clinic. Mediterranean Diet: A heart-healthy eating plan. Web. 2019. Available at: https://www.mayoclinic.org/healthy-lifestyle/nutrition-and-healthy-eating/in-depth/mediterranean-diet/art-20047801. Accessed January 9, 2021.
4. U.S. Department of Health and Human Services and U.S. Department of Agriculture. 2015–2020 dietary guidelines for Americans. 8th edition. 2015. Available at: http://health.gov/dietaryguidelines/2015/guidelines/. Accessed January 8, 2021.
5. Grundy SM, Stone NJ, Bailey AL, et al. 2018 AHA/ACC/AACVPR/AAPA/ABC/ACPM/ADA/AGS/APhA/ASPC/NLA/PCNA guideline on the management of blood cholesterol: executive summary: a report of the American College of Cardiology/American Heart Association Task Force on Clinical Practice Guidelines [published correction appears in Circulation. 2019 Jun 18;139(25):e1178-e1181]. Circulation 2019;139(25):e1046–81.
6. Whelton PK, Carey RM, Aronow WS, et al. 2017 ACC/AHA/AAPA/ABC/ACPM/AGS/APhA/ASH/ASPC/NMA/PCNA guideline for the prevention, detection, evaluation, and management of high blood pressure in adults: a report of the American College of Cardiology/American Heart Association Task Force on Clinical

Practice Guidelines [published correction appears in Hypertension. 2018 Jun;71(6):e140-e144]. Hypertension 2018;71(6):e13–115.

7. Mayo Clinic. DASH Diet: healthy eating to lower your blood pressure. Web. 2019. Available at: https://www.mayoclinic.org/healthy-lifestyle/nutrition-and-healthy-eating/in-depth/dash-diet/art-20048456. Accessed January 9, 2021.

8. Vane JR, Botting RM. The mechanism of action of aspirin. Thromb Res 2003; 110(5–6):255–8.

9. Raber I, McCarthy CP, Vaduganathan M, et al. The rise and fall of aspirin in the primary prevention of cardiovascular disease. Lancet 2019;393(10186):2155–67.

10. Gelbenegger G, Postula M, Pecen L, et al. Aspirin for primary prevention of cardiovascular disease: a meta-analysis with a particular focus on subgroups. BMC Med 2019;17(1):198.

11. Aspirin for the prevention of cardiovascular disease: U.S. preventive services task force recommendation statement. Ann Intern Med 2009;150(6):396.

12. ASCVD Risk Estimator +. Acc.org. Available at: http://tools.acc.org/ASCVD-Risk-Estimator-Plus/#!/calculate/estimate/. Accessed January 13, 2021.

13. Recommendation: Aspirin use to prevent cardiovascular disease and colorectal cancer: Preventive medication. Uspreventiveservicestaskforce.org. Available at: https://www.uspreventiveservicestaskforce.org/uspstf/draft-update-summary/aspirin-use-to-prevent-cardiovascular-disease-and-colorectal-cancer-preventive-medication. Accessed January 13, 2021.

14. Manson JE, Cook NR, Lee I-M, et al. Marine n-3 fatty acids and prevention of cardiovascular disease and cancer. N Engl J Med 2019;380(1):23–32.

15. ASCEND Study Collaborative Group, Bowman L, Mafham M, et al. Effects of n-3 fatty acid supplements in diabetes mellitus. N Engl J Med 2018;379(16):1540–50.

16. Yokoyama M, Origasa H, Matsuzaki M, et al. Effects of eicosapentaenoic acid on major coronary events in hypercholesterolaemic patients (JELIS): a randomised open-label, blinded endpoint analysis. Lancet 2007;369(9567):1090–8.

17. Tummala R, Ghosh RK, Jain V, et al. Fish oil and cardiometabolic diseases: Recent updates and controversies. Am J Med 2019;132(10):1153–9.

18. Piepoli MF, Hoes AW, Brotons C, et al. Main messages for primary care from the 2016 European Guidelines on cardiovascular disease prevention in clinical practice. Eur J Gen Pract 2018;24(1):51–6.

19. Siscovick DS, Barringer TA, Fretts AM, et al. Omega-3 polyunsaturated fatty acid (fish oil) supplementation and the prevention of clinical cardiovascular disease: a science advisory from the American Heart Association. Circulation 2017;135(15):e867–84.

20. Hecht H, Blaha MJ, Berman DS, et al. Clinical indications for coronary artery calcium scoring in asymptomatic patients: Expert consensus statement from the Society of Cardiovascular Computed Tomography. J Cardiovasc Comput Tomogr 2017;11(2):157–68.

21. Recommendation: Statin use for the primary prevention of cardiovascular disease in adults: Preventive medication. Uspreventiveservicestaskforce.org. Available at: https://www.uspreventiveservicestaskforce.org/uspstf/recommendation/statin-use-in-adults-preventive-medication. Accessed January 13, 2021.

22. Blaha MJ, Mortensen MB, Kianoush S, et al. Coronary artery calcium scoring. JACC Cardiovasc Imaging 2017;10(8):923–37.

23. Goff DC Jr, Lloyd-Jones DM, Bennett G, et al. 2013 ACC/AHA guideline on the assessment of cardiovascular risk: a report of the American College of Cardiology/American Heart Association Task Force on Practice Guidelines. Circulation 2014;129(25 Suppl 2):S49–73.

24. Nasir K, Bittencourt MS, Blaha MJ, et al. Implications of coronary artery calcium testing among statin candidates according to American College Of Cardiology/ American Heart Association Cholesterol Management Guidelines. J Am Coll Cardiol 2015;66(15):1657–68.

25. US Preventive Services Task Force, Curry SJ, Krist AH, et al. Screening for cardiovascular disease risk with electrocardiography: US preventive services task force recommendation statement. JAMA 2018;319(22):2308–14.

26. Siu AL, U S Preventive Services Task Force. Screening for abnormal blood glucose and type 2 diabetes mellitus: U.S. preventive services task force recommendation statement. Ann Intern Med 2015;163(11):861–8.

Obesity Prevention

Stephanie Jalaba, MMS, PA-C[a],*, Heather Trudeau, MPAS, PA-C[b],
Scott Carlson, DO, MPH[c]

KEYWORDS

• Obesity • Prevention • Nutrition • Exercise • Diet

KEY POINTS

• Given the current trajectory of obesity rates, prevention is paramount to the future health of society.
• Guidelines for healthy dietary patterns and adequate exercise are the current cornerstones of obesity-prevention efforts.
• Obesity-prevention strategies should be holistic, exploring alternate contributors such as weight bias and stress.

INTRODUCTION/HISTORY

Through much of human history, weight gain was seen as a sign of health and prosperity. In the 19th century, scholars began to debunk this age-old belief with discoveries such as fat storage in cells and publication of the first diet book, *Letter on Corpulence Addressed to the Public* by Mr. W. Banting. It was not until the early 20th century that an association between obesity and increased death rate was noted.[1] Fast forward to June 1997, The World Health Organization (WHO) Consultation on Obesity met in Geneva after 2 years of preparation by over 100 world experts to review the current epidemiology of obesity and create the framework for public health policies and programs that would aim to improve prevention and management of obesity.[1] It was at this time that obesity gained widespread recognition as an "epidemic."

DEFINITION OF OBESITY

Obesity is recognized as a chronic disease which occurs when excess fat accumulation increases the risk of poor health.[2] Although simply defined, obesity is a complex, multifactorial disease process that poses a significant threat to our population. The

[a] Department of PA Medicine, Michigan State University College of Osteopathic Medicine, 909 Wilson Road, West Fee B401A, E Lansing, MI 48824, USA; [b] Department of PA Medicine, Michigan State University College of Osteopathic Medicine, 909 Wilson Road, West Fee B401B, E Lansing, MI 48824, USA; [c] Department of PA Medicine, Michigan State University College of Osteopathic Medicine, 909 Wilson Road, West Fee B419A, E. Lansing, MI 48824, USA
* Corresponding author.
E-mail address: jalabast@msu.edu

Physician Assist Clin 7 (2022) 43–58
https://doi.org/10.1016/j.cpha.2021.07.004
2405-7991/22/© 2021 Elsevier Inc. All rights reserved.
physicianassistant.theclinics.com

interaction of genetic, biologic, metabolic, behavioral, environmental, and socioeconomic factors all potentially contributing to obesity highlights just how complex it is.[3] Obesity has been linked to an increased risk for the development of multiple different noncommunicable diseases (NCDs), notably cardiovascular disease (CVD), diabetes, musculoskeletal disorders, and several different cancers.[4] Moreover, obesity independently increases risk for almost all CVD risk factors including hypertension, dyslipidemia, metabolic syndrome, and type 2 diabetes mellitus (T2DM).[5] Obesity contributes to decreased life expectancy,[3] and furthermore, it is responsible for over 4 million deaths each year.[2] In addition, people with obesity experience diminished psychological health because of stigmas and weight biases.[3] Adding to the numerous other public health challenges we face as a nation, the medical care costs of obesity in the United States range from 147 billion to nearly 210 billion dollars per year.[5] Arguably, one of the most important defining factors of obesity is that it is preventable. In fact, obesity is one of the leading causes of preventable deaths in the United States.[5] Despite well-established knowledge of the importance of prevention, as well as the many targeted efforts aimed at prevention, obesity remains a problem of epidemic proportion across much of the globe.

PREVALENCE/INCIDENCE OF OBESITY

The prevalence of obesity around the world has nearly tripled between 1975 and 2016. In 2016, 39% of adults in the global population were classified as overweight and 13% were classified as obese. This equates to nearly 650 million obese adults. In 2019, the estimate of children younger than 5 years who were overweight or obese reached 38.2 million.[2]

In the United States, the age-adjusted rate of obesity among all adults was 42.4% in 2017 to 2018 as compared to 30.5% in 1999 to 2000, with prevalence of severe obesity reaching 9.2%, almost double what it was in 1999 to 2000 (**Fig. 1**).[6] When the overweight population is factored in, 74% of adults in the United States are overweight or obese.[7] Obesity rates in children and adolescents aged 2 to 19 years increase with each age group, starting as high as 13.9% in 2- to 5-year-olds and increasing to 18.4% in 6- to 11-year-olds and 20.6% in 12- to 19-year-olds (**Fig. 2**).[8]

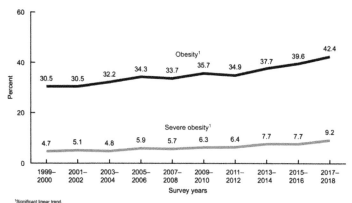

Fig. 1. Trends in age-adjusted obesity and severe obesity prevalence among adults aged 20 years and older: United States, 1999-2000 through 2017-2018.[6] (*Data from* NCHS Data Brief No. 360: Prevalence of Obesity and Severe Obesity Among Adults: United States, 2017-2018, Figure 4).

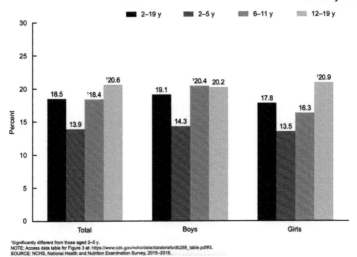

Fig. 2. Prevalence of obesity among youth aged 2-19 years, by sex and age: United States, 2015-2016.[8] (*Data from* NCHS Data Brief No. 288: Prevalence of Obesity Among Adults and Youth: United States, 2015-2016, Figure 3.)

Differences in obesity rates are seen among various sexes, age groups, races, ethnic groups, and other groupings. For example, as of 2017 to 2018, non-Hispanic black adult women had the highest prevalence of obesity (56.9%) compared to all other groups in the United States, including Hispanic women (43.7%), non-Hispanic white women (39.8%), and non-Hispanic Asian women (17.2%). Non-Hispanic black adult women obesity rates are also significantly higher than those of Hispanic adult men (45.7%), non-Hispanic white males (44.7%), non-Hispanic black males (41.1%), and non-Hispanic Asian men (17.5%).[6] Among children aged 2 to 19 years, Hispanic boys had the highest rates of obesity (28.0%) in 2015 to 2016. This was significantly different from all non-Hispanic black children (22.0%), non-Hispanic white children (14.1%), and non-Hispanic Asian children (11.0%).[8]

Perhaps one of the most eye-opening differences is seen among socioeconomic status groups in varying countries. Obesity was previously a problem only widely recognized in mostly higher income countries, but it has since expanded indiscriminately across the globe.[9] Many low- to middle-income countries face a "double burden" when undernutrition and subsequent emerging overnutrition are coupled together.[10] This "double burden" refers to the presence of both obesity and underweight in the same populations, communities, or even families and emphasizes the consequences of poor nutrition in early life.[11] With the vast majority of overweight or obese children now living in developing countries, this yet again highlights the importance of prevention.[2]

METHODS OF PREVENTION

Despite all that is known about obesity, controversy exists regarding the relative importance of certain contributing factors such as caloric intake, type of calories consumed, and caloric expenditure. Coupled with genetic, biologic, and behavioral factors, therein lies controversy concerning the most effective methods to target in the prevention of obesity. Concepts such as the "obesity paradox," which describes a metabolically healthy obese phenotype, further complicate the preventative approach.

MULTIMODAL APPROACH

Research and efforts throughout history have proven that although some factors contribute to obesity more than others, there is no single intervention that is going to adequately contribute to the sustainable prevention of obesity. Thus, it is important to consider a holistic approach in prevention efforts. This starts with simply recognizing obesity as a chronic disease. Sharma and Ramos Salas[12] suggest that lack of recognition of obesity as a chronic disease can negatively influence access to evidence-based prevention and treatment.

As with much of medicine, the "one-size-fits-all" approach to tackling obesity fails to consider the many different potential contributing factors and the realistic translation to sustainability. One of the many overall goals for prevention of weight gain is a chronic energy balance, which occurs when calories consumed through eating and drinking equal the calories burned with physical activity.[13] Because of this, the most popular targets for obesity prevention are undoubtedly nutrition and physical activity. However, successful prevention must incorporate additional tactics. It is well established that obesity is a complex interplay of many factors beyond diet and exercise. Simplistic obesity-prevention strategies that focus on healthy eating and physical activity alone can promote the weight-biased narrative that obesity can be controlled solely through individual efforts. This article will explore best strategies for nutrition and physical activity and also highlight additional factors to consider in individualized obesity-prevention strategies.

NUTRITION

Both quality and quantity of nutrition have proven to be important drivers of the energy imbalance that leads to obesity.[5] The ninth edition of the *Dietary Guidelines for Americans, 2020 to 2025* was published in December of 2020.[7] This guideline, published by the United States Department of Agriculture (USDA) and the Department of Health and Human Services (HHS) aims to benefit everyone, regardless of their race, age, ethnicity, socioeconomic status, or health status through inclusivity of scientific data representative of diverse populations.[7] The *Dietary Guidelines for Americans* focuses on health promotion and disease prevention by emphasizing dietary patterns in a lifespan approach. The basis for this approach lies in the consistent scientific evidence demonstrating that healthy dietary patterns are associated with beneficial outcomes for all-cause mortality, overweight and obesity, T2DM, bone health, CVD, and certain cancers.[7] This guideline recognizes that caloric needs change over time and provides guidance specific to each stage of life, including pregnancy and lactation.[7] The emphasis on dietary patterns rather than on single-food groups is consistent with The Obesity Society/American Heart Association/American College of Cardiology 2013 guidelines.[7,14] Overall, dietary recommendations of the *Dietary Guidelines for Americans, 2020 to 2025* stand consistent with the Dietary Approach to Stop Hypertension (DASH) diet and Mediterranean-style diets with emphasis on vegetables, fruits, legumes, nuts, whole grains, and low-fat dairy and favoring fish or poultry over red meat, although there are slight differences.[5,7,15] Mediterranean diets and the DASH diet have long been praised for their success in promoting weight loss with such feasibility that they avoid the typical "rebound" after weight loss and consistently reducing CVD risk factors.[5,7,14,15] The relative ease of incorporating these diets into a long-term strategy makes them more amenable to use for prevention purposes. Other "fad" diets such as ketogenic diets have proven effective in weight loss but have questionable safety and sustainability.[16] More robust studies are needed to examine the safety and long-term effects of these diets, in addition to their potential role in obesity prevention.

When it comes to quantity, the age-old saying "everything in moderation" still stands. Diets such as the DASH diet and Mediterranean-style diets contain serving size and portion recommendations aimed at overall health recommendations. The latest edition of the *Dietary Guidelines for Americans* includes a call to action to "make every bite count" by choosing nutrient-dense foods and staying within calorie limits.[7]

AGE	Males			Females		
	Sedentary[a]	Moderately Active[b]	Active[c]	Sedentary[a]	Moderately Active[b]	Active[c]
2	1,000	1,000	1,000	1,000	1,000	1,000
3	1,000	1,400	1,400	1,000	1,200	1,400
4	1,200	1,400	1,600	1,200	1,400	1,400
5	1,200	1,400	1,600	1,200	1,400	1,600
6	1,400	1,600	1,800	1,200	1,400	1,600
7	1,400	1,600	1,800	1,200	1,600	1,800
8	1,400	1,600	2,000	1,400	1,600	1,800
9	1,600	1,800	2,000	1,400	1,600	1,800
10	1,600	1,800	2,200	1,400	1,800	2,000
11	1,800	2,000	2,200	1,600	1,800	2,000
12	1,800	2,200	2,400	1,600	2,000	2,200
13	2,000	2,200	2,600	1,600	2,000	2,200
14	2,000	2,400	2,800	1,800	2,000	2,400
15	2,200	2,600	3,000	1,800	2,000	2,400
16	2,400	2,800	3,200	1,800	2,000	2,400
17	2,400	2,800	3,200	1,800	2,000	2,400
18	2,400	2,800	3,200	1,800	2,000	2,400
19-20	2,600	2,800	3,000	2,000	2,200	2,400
21-25	2,400	2,800	3,000	2,000	2,200	2,400
26-30	2,400	2,600	3,000	1,800	2,000	2,400
31-35	2,400	2,600	3,000	1,800	2,000	2,200
36-40	2,400	2,600	2,800	1,800	2,000	2,200
41-45	2,200	2,600	2,800	1,800	2,000	2,200
46-50	2,200	2,400	2,800	1,800	2,000	2,200
51-55	2,200	2,400	2,800	1,600	1,800	2,200
56-60	2,200	2,400	2,600	1,600	1,800	2,200

Fig. 3. Estimated calorie needs per day, by age, sex, and physical activity level, aged 2 years and older.[7] [a] Sedentary means a lifestyle that includes only the physical activity of independent living. [b] Moderately active means a lifestyle that includes physical activity equivalent to walking about 1.5 to 3 miles per day at 3 to 4 miles per hour, in addition to the activities of independent living. [c] Active means a lifestyle that includes physical activity equivalent to walking more than 3 miles per day at 3 to 4 miles per hour, in addition to the activities of independent living. (*Data from* Dietary Guidelines for Americans, 2020-2025 report, Appendix 2, Table A2-2.)

In order to maintain chronic energy balance, caloric recommendations (quantity) can be targeted at the individual level, based on activity level (**Fig. 3**).[7]

In addition to quantity, quality must be considered with regard to nutritional sources. Specific recommendations from the *Dietary Guidelines for Americans* include replacing most refined grains with whole grains, decreasing sodium, decreasing saturated fat, consuming fewer calories from added sugars, and replacing these calories with more varied vegetable choices, seafood, plant proteins, and low-fat dairy.[7] Data pooled from 3 population cohort studies in middle-aged and older adults illustrate additional considerations when choosing quality foods, demonstrating consistently less weight gain with intake of lower glycemic index and higher fiber vegetables and whole grains, nuts, and fruits across a 4-year follow-up period.[5] On the contrary, added sugars and sugar-sweetened beverages are identified as consistent dietary features associated with obesity.[17] In response to growing concerns with the association of added sugars and obesity, the *Dietary Guidelines for Americans* recommended reducing added sugar intake to less than 10% of total caloric intake in the 2015 report, and this stayed consistent in the 2020 to 2025 report.[7]

PHYSICAL ACTIVITY

Healthy physical activity practices, similar to nutrition, are important to instill starting at a young age to optimize preventative efforts. Benefits of physical activity on overall health are well established. Just one session of moderate-to-vigorous physical activity can improve insulin sensitivity, reduce blood pressure, reduce anxiety, improve cognition, and more.[18] Furthermore, regular physical activity helps maintain stable weight over time; improves weight status in children, adolescents, and adults; and can even reduce the risk of excess weight gain and incidence of obesity.[18] Moderate or vigorous aerobic activity is emphasized for the maintenance of weight, although muscle-strengthening also offers some benefit.

Despite efforts such as *Healthy People 2020*,[19] the current activity level of most Americans is insufficient, putting them at risk for chronic disease and other health issues.[18] There has been slight improvement in activity level among American adults, yet only 26% of men and 19% of women meet the guidelines set forth by the HHS and USDA.[18] As a complement to the *Dietary Guidelines for Americans*, the HHS and USDA have also developed the *Physical Activity Guidelines for Americans*, of which the 2nd edition was published in 2018.[18] The focus of these guidelines is disease prevention and health promotion in children, adolescents, and adults through different types of physical activity: aerobic, muscle-strengthening, bone-strengthening, balance, and flexibility. In this report, the committee recommends the following specific levels of activity:

- Children and adolescents aged 6 to 17 years should do 60 minutes or more of moderate-to-vigorous physical activity daily, incorporating aerobic, muscle-strengthening, and bone-strengthening activities, each at least 3 times weekly.
- Adults should do at least 150 minutes – 300 minutes per week of moderate-intensity, OR 75 minutes – 150 minutes per week of vigorous-intensity aerobic activity, OR an equivalent combination of both, adding in muscle-strengthening activities at least 2 days per week.

Unfortunately, it is not just as simple as incorporating the appropriate amount of physical activity into one's lifestyle. Sedentary behavior, classified as any waking behavior with energy expenditure less than or equal to 1.5 metabolic equivalents,[18] has recently been brought to light as a key player in public health problems. It is estimated that children and adults spend about 7.7 hours per day being sedentary.[18] The strong relationship between sedentary behaviors and all-cause mortality is clear,[18] but evidence regarding the specific link between sedentary behavior and obesity when controlled for physical activity is inconclusive and lacking.[5] It appears that the risk of all-cause mortality may be mitigated with physical activity. High volumes of moderate-to-vigorous physical activity appear to remove the excess risk of all-cause mortality associated with high volumes of sitting.[18] Given the aforementioned findings, more research in this area is prudent to providing the public with the best possible obesity-prevention measures.

OVERVIEW OF WEIGHT BIAS, STIGMA, AND DISCRIMINATION

The spotlight on social injustices has made society increasingly aware of the far-reaching negative effects of biases and marginalizing groups of people, which also apply to those with obesity. Unfortunately, many individuals with obesity are no strangers to bias, stigma, marginalization, or even discrimination, not only from society in general, but also from health care providers alike.

Weight bias is defined as "negative weight-related attitudes, beliefs, assumptions, and judgements toward individuals who are overweight and obese."[20] These negative biases may stem from generalizations that individuals with obesity are personally responsible for their condition because they are sedentary, lack exercise, or have poor eating habits. These generalizations lead to weight stigma, which is defined as "social devaluation and denigration of individuals because of their excess body weight."[21] The negative attitudes toward obese individuals do not stop at bias. These individuals can also experience discrimination. Weight bias and discrimination can manifest in multiple aspects of life, including employment, health care, educational settings, interpersonal relationships, and even in the media.[22] With the widespread prevalence of weight bias and discrimination in society, individuals with obesity can begin to engage in self-blame and self-directed weight stigma.[21] For this reason, weight bias can have far-reaching physical and mental health consequences on obese individuals, such as poor body image, social isolation, depression, anxiety, substance use, lower self-esteem, avoidance of physical activity, maladaptive eating patterns, stress-induced pathophysiologic changes, and avoidance of medical care.[21,23]

A systematic review by Spahlholz and colleagues[22] found the prevalence of weight discrimination in adults ranging from 19% to 42%, with the highest rates seen in those with higher body mass index (BMI) values and in women. Weight/height discrimination has been cited as the third most common type of discrimination among women and the fourth most common type of discrimination among all adults.[24]

WEIGHT BIAS IN THE HEALTH CARE SETTING

It is safe to assume that health care providers do not intend to treat obese patients with bias, yet the occurrence of this phenomenon is remarkable. According to a study by Puhl and Brownell[25] that surveyed over 2400 women with obesity, 69% reported stigmatization by physicians. Many studies show no difference in the attitudes displayed toward different genders or races; however, women tend to internalize weight bias more than men.[26] Bias has been observed across multiple layers of the health care team, including primary care providers, endocrinologists, cardiologists, nurses, dietitians, mental health professionals, medical trainees, and researchers.[21]

Weight bias can negatively influence many aspects of care for patients with obesity. Research suggests that medical professionals who are weight-biased may spend less time and provide less health education,[27] demonstrate less respect,[28] and demonstrate less emotional rapport.[29] Patients with reported weight bias can experience poor treatment outcomes, are more likely to avoid future care, and may even be less likely to receive age-appropriate cancer screenings.[21] Finally, it has been suggested that the negative consequences of weight bias on the individual may be more harmful than obesity itself.[30]

PREVENTING WEIGHT BIAS IN OBESITY

Addressing weight bias and stigma can influence overall obesity-prevention efforts. Eliminating weight bias from practice is not straightforward, however. There are multiple considerations that must be addressed over time to enact lasting change. An international, multidisciplinary group of obesity experts published a joint international consensus statement in March 2020 with recommendations to eliminate weight bias.[21] This statement includes a call to action for all stakeholders to take a pledge to end weight stigma and discrimination. The call to action highlights the unproven assumption that obesity is a personal responsibility and the more evidence-based stance that biological, environmental, and genetic factors all contribute to obesity.[21] Recommendations for providers include treating overweight or obese patients respectfully, avoiding stereotypical language, and supporting both educational initiatives aimed at eliminating weight bias and initiatives to eliminate discrimination based on weight.[21]

Evidence suggests that simply having a conversation about obesity can lead to weight loss.[26] Although it seems simple, apprehension to have these conversations is reported from both health care providers and obese patients.[26] Some of the apprehension may stem from concern of offending the patient, receiving a negative reaction, or damaging a sound relationship with a patient.[26] In one study by Berg and colleagues,[31] 74% of pediatricians surveyed were not worried about offending families by talking about weight, but only 59% felt that families wanted it discussed, and most felt that counseling has poor results. Improving communication and using appropriate language to discuss obesity and reduce stigma are the focus of the recent joint consensus statement *The Importance of Language Engagement Between Health-care Professionals and People Living with Obesity*.[26] Recommended conversation features include the use of person-centered language, the use of language that is free from judgment or negative connotation, avoidance of combative language or humor, sticking to the evidence, avoiding blame, and avoiding making assumptions.[26] Beyond lapses in language and communication, many providers in preventative or general practice are perceived by obese patients as lacking the training to offer effective resources or weight-management recommendations.[32] Furthermore, the language of public health campaigns can often be perceived as biased. Puhl and colleagues found[33] that obese participants were less likely to comply with public health media campaigns with stigmatizing messages. These participants found public health campaigns that focused on making healthy behavioral changes without referencing body weight or using the word "obesity" to be the most positive and motivating.[33]

In addition to the social environment, the physical environment of a medical facility can unintentionally promote weight bias and become a barrier to seeking medical care among obese populations.[32] Waiting rooms and examination rooms may be inappropriately equipped with gowns, examination tables, chairs, and blood pressure cuffs that cannot accommodate larger body sizes. In addition, obese individuals have cited not wanting to get weighed, fear of exposing their bodies, and undressing in health care offices as reasons they avoid seeking care.[32] Studies have shown that a higher BMI is associated with a decrease in utilization of health care services.[32] This avoidance could lead to unaddressed progressive obesity-related comorbidities and complications and hinder the prevention and management of obesity.[32]

STRESS AND WEIGHT GAIN

Oftentimes, it is necessary to examine potential contributing factors to obesity beyond what may be considered a "normal" workup. Chronic stress, posttraumatic stress disorder (PTSD), or history of mental, physical, and/or sexual abuse all may potentially contribute to weight gain.[34,35] Evidence has shown that this is primarily mediated by an increase in the stress hormone cortisol, which plays a role in obesity.[34] Cortisol increases the body's appetite for energy-dense or "comfort" foods and can eventually cause abdominal adiposity.[36] In acute stress events, corticotropin-releasing hormone causes acute appetite suppression, but in short time, the production of glucocorticoids, including cortisol, causes stimulation of appetite.[34] The body transiently adapts by triggering several physiologic reactions, including insulin resistance. Beyond acute effects, prolonged and repeated cortisol release may cause long-term physiologic dysregulation.[37] The chronic effects of stress can lead to several different metabolic and neurobiological changes, of which the downstream effects can be particularly damaging to overall health. Although a full discussion of these changes is beyond the scope of this article, two metabolic changes caused by chronic stress worth mentioning are an increase in adipocyte development and increased glucocorticoid receptor activity. These factors increase the risk of abdominal adiposity, which is an independent risk factor for CVD and is also known to negatively affect several other CVD risk factors including blood pressure, plasma lipoproteins, and insulin resistance.[37] In chronic stress, both a dysregulated stress system and behavioral habits can lead to obesity, metabolic syndrome, T2DM, and CVD.[38] Decreased sleep, intake of foods with high glycemic index, chronic pain, and excess alcohol use can all enhance the body's stress response.[34]

A novel technique for measuring long-term retrospective cortisol levels has been discovered in human scalp hair sampling, hair cortisol concentration (HCC).[39] The correlation between HCC and certain mental states has been examined in several studies.[34] Depression and obesity tend to co-occur in many individuals, suggesting the correlation of HCC and mental state may provide some insight into the correlation of obesity and cortisol.[40] In general, those with chronic perceived stress tend to have higher HCC levels.[34] In connection with earlier discussion, obese individuals who experience weight discrimination were found to have 33% higher HCC levels than obese individuals who did not experience weight discrimination, and this was even more pronounced in the severely obese population.[41]

TARGETING THE PEDIATRIC POPULATION

Overweight and obesity are associated with significant comorbidities in childhood such as prediabetes and T2DM, prehypertension and hypertension, sleep apnea, nonalcoholic fatty liver disease, and polycystic ovary syndrome.[42] When considering the potential implications of pediatric obesity later in life and the steady increase in obesity prevalence statistics with increasing age, this is perhaps the best population to target preventative efforts at, although prevention across the lifespan is undeniably important. For this reason, it is important that parents have an accurate understanding of their child's weight and the implications it could have on their health. Research has shown that greater than 75% of parents with an overweight child report that they were never made aware of this.[43] This could partially be attributable to lack of identification on the provider's end. In one study, almost all primary care physicians surveyed reported measuring height and weight (99%) and visually assessing for overweight status (97%) at almost every visit. However, only about half of the respondents (52%) used BMI percentile for children older than 2 years.[44] This is detrimental considering the poor reliability of visual assessment. One study by Berg and colleagues[31] examined the performance of physician assistant students and recent physician assistant graduates in estimating BMI categorization of young children by visual assessment. The results were consistent with studies examining other medical professionals' performance in that visual assessments alone are unreliable, especially for classifying overweight and obese children.[31]

Specific guidelines aimed at obesity prevention have been established in the pediatric population. The *Endocrine Society Clinical Practice Guideline on Assessment, Treatment, and Prevention of Pediatric Obesity* was published in 2017.[42] Recommendations for prevention of obesity include avoiding consumption of calorie-dense, nutrient-poor foods, encouraging the consumption of whole fruits rather than fruit juices, engaging in at least 20 minutes (optimally 60 minutes) of vigorous physical activity at least 5 days per week, fostering healthy sleep patterns, and balancing unavoidable screen time with increased physical activity. Furthermore, the guidelines suggest that clinicians aim obesity-prevention efforts at the whole family rather than the individual patient, assess family function and make referrals to decrease stressors where necessary, use community engagement and school-based programs, use comprehensive behavior-changing interventions, and encourage breast-feeding in infants.[42] Although most of these recommendations are straightforward, prescribing and monitoring of these recommendations do not come without challenges. In addition to patient and family adherence and follow-up, poor reimbursement for these services and inadequate national and international recognition of the value of addressing obesity prevention pose additional barriers.[42]

EARLY LIFE STRESS AND METABOLIC EFFECTS

The effects of stress are particularly damaging in the fetal through adolescent stages of life.[38] Childhood adversity, sometimes the cause of PTSD, has been found to impact central obesity even when other risk factors are controlled for.[45] Childhood and adolescent stress lead to particularly worsened central obesity, insulin resistance, and metabolic syndrome.[46] The amygdala, hippocampus, and mesocorticolimbic system, all in development during fetal, child, and adolescent years are responsible for stress regulation and are particularly vulnerable to the effects of stress in these years.[38] Additionally, chronically altered cortisol secretion in childhood can lead to early-onset obesity and metabolic syndrome, among many other effects. It has been postulated that better understanding the effects of stress mechanisms in early life could lead to more effective prevention of obesity. Recognizing real or perceived stress as a variable of metabolic risk might lead to improvements in both prevention and intervention of early life stressors and, in turn, their damaging consequences such as obesity and metabolic syndrome.[38]

Adverse childhood experiences (ACEs) are potentially traumatic events that occur in childhood before the age of 18 years. These events may include experiencing violence, abuse, or neglect; witnessing violence in the home or community; having a family member attempt or die by suicide; or unsafe or unstable living environments.[47] A growing body of evidence has linked ACEs to mental illness, substance misuse, and chronic health problems including obesity in adulthood.[47–49] A 2014 meta-analysis by Hemmingsson and colleagues[48] found that adults who were exposed to childhood abuse (physical, emotional, or sexual) were significantly more likely to develop obesity and showed a positive dose-response association between abuse severity and obesity risk. Many potential mechanisms for this increased risk were discussed, including elevated cortisol levels due to chronic stress.[48] Williamson and colleagues[49] suggest that preventing child abuse may decrease adult obesity.

ACEs are thought to be preventable and are common, with 61% of surveyed adults reporting at least one type of ACE.[47] Questionnaires such as the Behavioral Risk Factor Surveillance System Ace Module can be used by clinicians in adults to identify ACEs that a patient may have experienced in childhood (**Box 1**).[47,50] During visits, providers have the opportunity to elicit a history of child abuse (mental, physical, or sexual), adversity (poverty, homeless, food insecure, frequent moves, loss of one or two parents), or PTSD (witnessing or experiencing a major life event such as a car crash, seeing a murder, kidnapped, and so forth). In these types of events, early intervention in family dynamics through utilization of social services and enhanced family support may be essential to optimizing overall health and wellness.

DISCUSSION

In today's medical climate, clinicians are increasingly pressed for time, allowing less opportunity for discussion of crucial issues such as obesity prevention. Obesity prevention is a complex issue that requires a thorough examination of patient and family lifestyle and risk factors and a tailored approach to best suit each individual. Investing time in patient and family education and aiming to establish healthy behaviors and identify risk factors for obesity at an early age is crucial to changing the current trajectory of the obesity epidemic. Furthermore, beyond providing patients with the tools for success, there remain several factors that clinicians cannot necessarily control for such as genetic risks and environmental influences.

Box 1
Adverse childhood experience questionnaire[50]

1. Did you live with anyone who was depressed, mentally ill, or suicidal?

2. Did you live with anyone who was a problem drinker or alcoholic?

3. Did you live with anyone who used illegal street drugs or who abused prescription medications?

4. Did you live with anyone who served time or was sentenced to serve time in a prison, jail, or other correctional facility?

5. Were your parents separated or divorced?

6. How often did your parents or adults in your home ever slap, hit, kick, punch, or beat each other up?

7. Before age 18, how often did a parent in your home ever hit, beat, kick, or physically hurt you in any way? Do not include spanking.

8. How often did a parent or adult in your home ever swear at you, insult you, or put you down?

9. How often did anyone at least 5 years older than you or an adult ever touch you sexually?

10. How often did anyone at least 5 years older than you or an adult try to make you touch sexually?

11. How often did anyone at least 5 years older than you or an adult force you to have sex?

Data from National Center for Injury Prevention and Control, Division of Violence Prevention. Complete directions for the administration of this questionnaire can be found at: https://www. cdc.gov/violenceprevention/acestudy/pdf/BRFSS_Adverse_Module.pdf.

The many national and global public efforts aimed at physical activity and nutrition have proven ineffective up to this juncture, so perhaps it is time for a more holistic, individualized approach. Beyond nutrition and exercise, consideration may be given to additional factors such as reducing or eliminating weight bias to promote healthier and more trusting relationships between patients and providers and assessing stressors to understand how these may contribute to a patient's weight.

Patient education on such a sensitive topic must be approached with caution to avoid perception of bias or negativity by patients, which could potentially lead to self-blame, loss of motivation, avoidance of seeking care, or even depression. Providers must first recognize their own biases to provide effective care to this population.

Stress reduction is paramount but often an underappreciated tool for obesity prevention. Stress can lead to unhealthy behaviors in addition to the negative metabolic and neurobiological effects it causes. An assessment of stressors should be considered even at a young age, especially with the high reported rates of ACEs.

Around the world, the development of detrimental societal habits is contributing to overweight and obesity. Foods high in fat and sugars are prevalent; physical inactivity has largely increased over time because of sedentary forms of work, heavy reliance on technology for entertainment, and changing modes of transportation; racial and ethnic disparities continue to contribute to negative health outcomes on several levels; and fast-paced lifestyles continue to promote convenience over health. This is hardly an all-inclusive list.

In *Healthy People 2020* data published in 2014, two crucial targets of this national effort moved in a negative direction: obesity among children and adolescents and obesity among adults.[19] Obesity rates among children and adolescents increased from 16.1% to 16.9% rather than decreasing toward the target of 14.5%. Obesity rates among adults increased from 33.9% to 35.3%, moving away from the target of 30.5%.[19] As data for the 2020 targets are being compiled, the most devastating health crisis of our time has forced many into sedentary behaviors, lack of exercise routines, lack of fresh and healthy foods, lack of resources, and avoidance of medical care. One study published in May 2020 reported that roughly 22% of adults surveyed had gained 5 to 10 pounds in the initial months of the COVID-19 pandemic.[51] Lack of sleep, decreased physical activity, eating in response to stress, eating because of the appearance and smell of food, and snacking after dinner were all behaviors linked to weight gain during quarantine.[51] Given the ongoing nature of the pandemic, we are likely to see higher percentages of weight gain, less implementation of obesity prevention, and the lasting effects for many years to come.

SUMMARY

Given the steady climb in obesity rates through the years to epidemic levels and its link to multiple different NCDs, prevention of obesity is more critical than ever. Obesity is a complex, multifactorial chronic disease which necessitates a multifaceted, holistic approach to prevention. Although healthy diet and sufficient exercise typically serve as the cornerstone to prevention efforts, clinicians must shift to a more holistic assessment of contributing factors and consider individualized approaches. Strategies should aim for a realistic framework of sustainability over the lifespan. With the upward trend in obesity prevalence rates with increasing age, it is logical to target prevention efforts at the pediatric population with the hope that healthy behaviors established at an early age will be carried into adulthood. However, it should be emphasized that prevention is important regardless of age, and it may not always be an individual effort. In addition to provider training and resources, more research is needed to create evidence-based, holistic, and sustainable strategies for obesity prevention and to examine strategies for increasing compliance among the public. The effects of the currently poor trajectory of overweight and obesity are likely to be seen for decades to come. Shifting the paradigm of the current obesity-prevention narrative is of utmost importance, now more than ever.

CLINICS CARE POINTS

- Sources such as the *Dietary Guidelines for Americans* provide a realistic and sustainable framework for healthy eating patterns to help prevent overweight and obesity.
- The current activity level of most Americans is insufficient, and furthermore, sedentary behaviors are independently linked to all-cause mortality.
- Weight stigma and bias negatively affect obesity-prevention efforts, and the approach taken to discussing weight can make a significant difference in a patient's perception and compliance.
- Stress is often overlooked as a contributor to obesity, and the *Adverse Childhood Experience Questionnaire* is one tool to indirectly help prevent obesity by identifying stressors in childhood.

DISCLOSURE

The authors have nothing to disclose.

REFERENCES

1. World Health Organization. Obesity: preventing and managing the global epidemic. Report of a WHO Consultation of Obesity (WHO Technical Report Series 894). 2000. Available at: https://www.who.int/nutrition/publications/obesity/WHO_TRS_894/en/. Accessed November 30, 2020.
2. Obesity and Overweight. World Health Organization website. 2020. Available at: https://www.who.int/news-room/fact-sheets/detail/obesity-and-overweight. Accessed November 30, 2020.
3. Wharton S, Lau DCW, Vallis M, et al. Obesity in adults: a clinical practice guideline. CMAJ 2020;192(31):E875–91.
4. Chooi YC, Ding C, Magkos F. The epidemiology of obesity. Metabolism 2019; 92:6–10.
5. Lavie CJ, Laddu D, Arena R, et al. Healthy weight and obesity prevention: JACC health promotion series. J Am Coll Cardiol 2018;72(13):1506–31.
6. Hales CM, Carroll MD, Fryar CD, et al. US Department of Health and Human Services Centers for Disease Control and Prevention – National Center for Health Statistics. NCHS Data Brief, no 360: prevalence of obesity and severe obesity among adults: United States, 2017-2018. 2020. Available at: https://www.cdc.gov/nchs/data/databriefs/db360-h.pdf. Accessed December 1, 2020.
7. U.S. Department of Agriculture and U.S. Department of Health and Human Services. Dietary guidelines for Americans, 2020-2025. 9th edition 2020. USDA Publication #: USDA-FNS-2020-2025-DGA. HHS Publication #: HHS-ODPHP-2020-2025-01-DGA-A. Available at: https://www.dietaryguidelines.gov/sites/default/files/2020-12/Dietary_Guidelines_for_Americans_2020-2025.pdf. Accessed January 6, 2021.

8. Hales CM, Carroll MD, Fryar CD, et al. US Department of Health and Human Services Centers for Disease Control and Prevention – National Center for Health Statistics. NCHS Data Brief No. 288: prevalence of obesity among adults and youth: United states, 2015-2016. 2017. Available at: https://www.cdc.gov/nchs/data/databriefs/db288.pdf. Accessed December 1, 2020.

9. Seidell JC, Halberstadt J. The global burden of obesity and the challenges of prevention. Ann Nutr Metab 2015;66(suppl2):7–12.

10. Swinburn BA, Sacks G, Hall KD, et al. The global obesity pandemic: shaped by global drivers and local environments. Lancet 2011;378(9793):804–14.

11. World Health Organization. Guideline: assessing and managing children at primary health-care facilities to prevent overweight and obesity in the context of the double burden of malnutrition: updates for the integrated management of childhood illness (IMCI). 2017. Available at: https://www.ncbi.nlm.nih.gov/books/NBK487902/. Accessed November 30, 2020.

12. Sharma AM, Ramos Salas X. Obesity prevention and management strategies in canada: shifting paradigms and putting people first. Curr Obes Rep 2018;7(2):89–96.

13. Balance Food and Activity. National Heart, Lung, and Blood Institute website. 2013. Available at: https://www.nhlbi.nih.gov/health/educational/wecan/healthy-weight-basics/balance.htm. Accessed December 3, 2020.

14. Jensen MD, Ryan DH, Apovian CM, et al. 2013 AHA/ACC/TOS guideline for the management of overweight and obesity in adults: a report of the American college of cardiology/American heart association task force on practice guidelines and the obesity society. J Am Coll Cardiol 2014;63(25 Pt B):2985–3023.

15. Estruch R, Ros E, Salas-Salvado J, et al. Primary prevention of cardiovascular disease with a mediterranean diet. N Engl J Med 2013;368:1279–90.

16. O'Neill B, Raggi P. The ketogenic diet: pros and cons. Atherosclerosis 2020;292:119–26.

17. Arsenault BJ, Lamarche B, Despres JP. Targeting overconsumption of sugar-sweetened beverages vs. overall poor diet quality for cardiometabolic diseases risk prevention: place your bets! Nutrients 2017;9(6):600.

18. 2018 Physical Activity Guidelines Advisory Committee. Physical activity guidelines for americans. 2nd edition 2018. Available at: https://health.gov/sites/default/files/2019-09/Physical_Activity_Guidelines_2nd_edition.pdf. Accessed December 3, 2020.

19. US Department of Health and Human Services Office of Disease Prevention and Health Promotion. Healthy people 2020 leading health indicators: nutrition, physical activity, and obesity 2014. Available at: https://www.healthypeople.gov/sites/default/files/HP2020_LHI_Nut_PhysActiv.pdf. Accessed January 6, 2020.

20. Alberga AS, Russell-Mayhew S, von Ranson KM, et al. Weight bias: a call to action. J Eat Disord 2016;4:34.

21. Rubino F, Puhl RM, Cummings DE, et al. Joint international consensus statement for ending stigma of obesity. Nat Med 2020;26(4):485–97.

22. Spahlholz J, Baer N, König HH, et al. Obesity and discrimination - a systematic review and meta-analysis of observational studies. Obes Rev 2016 Jan;17(1):43–55.

23. World Health Organization: Regional Office for Europe. Weight Bias and Obesity Stigma: Considerations for the WHO European Region. 2017. Available at: https://www.euro.who.int/__data/assets/pdf_file/0017/351026/WeightBias.pdf. Accessed January 2, 2020.

24. Puhl R, Andreyeva T, Brownell K. Perceptions of weight discrimination: prevalence and comparison to race and gender discrimination in America. Int J Obes 2008;32:992–1000.
25. Puhl R, Brownell KD. Confronting and coping with weight stigma: an investigation of overweight and individuals with obesity. Obesity 2006;14:1802–15.
26. Albury C, Strain WD, Brocq SL, et al. The importance of language in engagement between health-care professionals and people living with obesity: a joint consensus statement. Lancet Diabetes Endocrinol 2020;8(5):447–55.
27. Phelan SM, Burgess DJ, Yeazel MW, et al. Impact of weight bias and stigma on quality of care and outcomes for patients with obesity. Obes Rev 2015;16(4):319–26.
28. Huizinga MM, Cooper LA, Bleich SN, et al. Physician respect for patients with obesity. J Gen Intern Med 2009;24(11):1236–9.
29. Gudzune KA, Beach MC, Roter DL, et al. Physicians build less rapport with obese patients. Obesity (Silver Spring) 2013;21(10):2146–52.
30. Sutin AR, Stephan Y, Terracciano A. Weight discrimination and risk of mortality. Psychol Sci 2015;26(11):1803–11.
31. Berg GM, Casper P, Ohlman E, et al. PA student assessment of body mass index in children using visual cues. J Am Acad Physician Assist 2017 Oct;30(10):37–41.
32. Nutter S, Russell-Mayhew S, Alberga AS, et al. Positioning of weight bias: moving towards social justice. J Obes 2016;2016(2):1–10.
33. Puhl RM, Himmelstein MS, Quinn DM. Internalizing weight stigma: prevalence and sociodemographic considerations in US adults. Obesity (Silver Spring) 2018;26(1):167–75.
34. Van der Valk ES, Savas M, van Rossum EFC. Stress and obesity: are there more susceptible individuals? Curr Obes Rep 2018;7:193–203.
35. Peckett AJ, Wright DC, Riddell MC. The effects of glucocorticoids on adipose tissue lipid metabolism. Metabolism 2011;60(11):1500–10.
36. Fardet L, Feve B. Systemic glucocorticoid therapy: a review of its metabolic and cardiovascular adverse events. Drugs 2014;74:1731–45.
37. Iob E, Steptoe A. Cardiovascular disease and hair cortisol: a novel biomarker of chronic stress. Curr Cardiol Rep 2019;21(10):116.
38. Farr OM, Sloan DM, Keane TM, Mantzoros CS. Stress-and PTSD-associated obesity and metabolic dysfunction: A growing problem requiring further research and novel treatments. Metabolism 2014;63(12):1463–8.
39. Noppe G, de Rijke YB, Dorst K, et al. LC-MS/MS-based method for long-term steroid profiling in human scalp hair. Clin Endocrinol 2015;83(2):162–6.
40. Milanesche Y, Simmons WK, van Rossum EFC, et al. Depression and obesity: evidence of shared biological mechanisms. Mol Psychiatry 2019;24(1):18–33.
41. Jackson SE, Kirschbaum C, Steptoe A. Perceived weight discrimination and chronic biochemical stress: A population-based study using cortisol in scalp hair. Obesity 2016;24(12):2515–21.
42. Styne DM, Arslanian SA, Connor EL, et al. Pediatric obesity – assessment, treatment, and prevention: an endocrine society clinical practice guideline. J Clin Endocrinol Metab 2017;102(3):709–57.
43. Brown CL, Perriin EM. Obesity prevention and treatment in primary care. Acad Pediatr 2018;18(7):736–45.
44. Klein JD, Sesselberg TS, Johnson MS, et al. Adoption of body mass index guidelines for screening and counseling in pediatric practice. Pediatrics 2010;125(2):265–72.

45. Davis CR, Dearing E, Usher N, et al. Detailed assessments of childhood adversity enhance prediction of central obesity independent of gender, race, adult psychosocial risk and health behaviors. Metabolism 2014;63(2):199–206.
46. Pervanidou P, Chrousos GP. Metabolic consequences of stress during childhood and adolescence. Metabolism 2012;61(5):611–9.
47. Adverse childhood experiences. Centers for Disease Control and Prevention website. 2020. Available at: https://www.cdc.gov/violenceprevention/aces/index.html. Accessed January 3, 2021.
48. Hemmingsson E, Johansson K, Reynisdottir S. Childhood abuse and adult obesity. Obes Rev 2014;15:882–93.
49. Williamson DF, Thompson TJ, Anda RF, et al. Body weight, obesity, and self-reported abuse in childhood external icon. Int J Obes 2002;26:1075–82.
50. Behavioral risk factor surveillance system ACE module questionnaire. Centers for Disease Control and Prevention website. Available at: https://www.cdc.gov/violenceprevention/acestudy/pdf/BRFSS_Adverse_Module.pdf. Accessed January 3, 2021.
51. Zeigler Z, Forbes B, Lopez B, et al. Self-quarantine and weight gain related risk factors during the COVID-19 pandemic. Obes Res Clin Pract 2020;14(3):210–6.

Under Pressure
Optimizing the Well-child Check in Children Aged 3 to 18 Years

Pollyanna Kabara, EdD, MS, PA-C

KEYWORDS

• Mental health • COVID-19 • Health disparity • Blood pressure • Screening

KEY POINTS

• Current circumstances pertaining to the pandemic and social climate create stress for patients, families, and providers.
• Primary care providers must assess multiple aspects of the patient's well-being, including vital signs and mental health; however, providers have limited time with patients during well child check.
• Two important screenings that should take place during well-child checks are blood pressure screening and mental health screening for depression and anxiety.
• There are many helpful resources to support patients and families/caregivers.

INTRODUCTION

Primary care providers have an opportunity to conduct assessments of mental health and provide support to promote mental health, in addition to traditional behavioral and developmental anticipatory guidance. The coronavirus disease 2019 (COVID-19) pandemic has affected children and their caregivers in a variety of ways, including negative health impact, loss of jobs and income, and childcare struggles. Children and parents are experiencing mental health challenges, and the mental health of parents tends to worsen as the economic situation worsens. Providers should screen for mental health concerns among all children, paying close attention to children whose families have experienced a negative impact related to the pandemic.[1]

Another important form of screening is an annual blood pressure. Children who have hypertension are more likely to have cardiovascular disease as adults.[2] The updated 2017 American Academy of Pediatrics Clinical Practice Guidelines stress that more children and adolescents than were previously identified could be classified as having hypertension because of revision of the inclusion and exclusion criteria of participants.[2]

Disclosure: The author has no financial conflicts of interest or funding sources to disclose.
Lakeside Pediatrics, 8600 75th Street, Ste 101, Kenosha, WI 53142, USA
E-mail address: pkabara@chw.org

Children aged 3 years and older should be screened for blood pressure abnormalities annually, and providers should use the updated blood pressure tables provided in the Clinical Practice Guidelines. The updated guidelines include tables that have been updated and are easier to use, and include static blood pressure thresholds for teenage patients that align with the revised adult blood pressure guidelines.[3]

BACKGROUND

Pediatric mental health concerns have significantly increased over the past 10 years.[4] These mental health concerns include depression, anxiety, and other behavioral disorders. In addition, there are more youth seeking treatment of self-harm and for psychiatric crises.[5] Approximately 20% of children in the United States between the ages of 3 and 17 years experience at least 1 form of mental health disorder, including attention-deficit/hyperactivity disorder, issues with behavior, and mood disorders.[6] Children who have mental health or behavioral disorders often continue to have mental health and behavioral disorders as adults.[7] Children and adolescents often do not receive appropriate assessment and treatment of mental health concerns, such as depression, anxiety, loneliness, social isolation, and suicide.[4]

Stress during times of crisis affects people in a cumulative fashion, resulting in outcomes that become worse over time. In addition, people experience similar stressors in different ways. Various factors, such as race, ethnicity, baseline health, socioeconomic status, and local and national resources, all have an impact on an individual's response to a stressful event.[8] The impact of the COVID-19 pandemic must be considered as pediatric patients are evaluated by their primary care providers.[8]

DISCUSSION

The COVID-19 pandemic has affected people of all ages in a variety of ways, including physically, emotionally, socially, and economically. Feelings of fear, anger, and boredom accompany states of feeling stressed, depressed, and anxious.[8] The public health precautions of social distancing and closures of schools affected more than 55 million children and adolescents.[9] School closure not only affects the children and adolescents but also has a significant impact on the caregiver because many scrambled to find childcare or transition to working from home while helping children with their schoolwork. Mental health may worsen in children and adolescents as the pandemic continues. Children and adolescents are not only affected by the social distancing and change in their school environment and social environments but they are also affected by the stressors that their families experience because of the pandemic. Economic stress and mental health concerns in caregivers may lead to increased child maltreatment.[9] The well-being of children, physically and emotionally, must be considered as policies are made in order to ensure that children receive the critical services that they need from the school environment. Many children rely on the breakfast and lunch programs at their schools as their primary source of nutrition.[9] Although many schools offer food pick-up services, families must have the means to travel to and from the school to pick up the food. In addition to the important nutrition programs that are offered at schools, many students receive mental health services, physical therapy, occupational therapy, and speech therapy at school.[9] School closures affected the manner in which these services were conducted. Adolescents in racial and ethnic minority groups often only receive mental health services through the school, and do not have immediate access to mental health services outside the school setting.[9]

Racial and ethnic health disparities have been accentuated by the COVID-19 pandemic, and patients from racial and/or ethnic minorities and socioeconomically disadvantaged patients are suffering from various aspects of the pandemic.[10] Goyal and colleagues'[10] study found that there are racial and ethnic disparities in the infection rates of COVID-19 in addition to the increased rate of COVID-19 infection in patients who are socioeconomically disadvantaged. They found that, in black patients, the higher rate of COVID-19 infection was significant, separate from socioeconomic status. One possible reason for the higher infection rates in minorities is that there is a higher proportion of minorities working as essential workers in service industries in which they must have face-to-face interaction with other people.[10] This study presents data that align with the data from studies conducted with adult patients with COVID-19. In addition to the higher infection rates among black patients, Hispanic patients also experience high rates of infection.[10] Goyal and colleagues[10] offer potential reasons for the high rate of COVID-19 in Hispanic patients, including use of public transportation, low rates of remote work, and high rates of childcare. Immigration status may also affect the infection rates of Hispanic children, as may the language barrier.[10] Racism affects many African American and Afro-Caribbean youth, and is a toxic stressor for these youth.[11] A recent study by Dr Lee Pachter, DO, FAAP, found that 85% of African American and Afro-Caribbean youth experienced discrimination. Dr Pachter separated African American and Afro-Caribbean youth instead of generalizing the youth as black in order to delineate unique experiences to each culture.[11] Dr Pachter's study found that African American and Afro-Caribbean youth who had multiple discriminatory experiences have a higher likelihood of mental health disorders as adults, in addition to having mental health disorders as youth.[11]

There are significant disparities pertaining to treatment of pediatric mental health disorders. Children and adolescents who are uninsured, from low-income families, and from minority racial and ethnic groups tend to have the least access to mental health treatment.[6] There are 3 levels of racism that affect these patients.[12] The first is institutionalized racism, which includes policies and practices that affect access.[12] The second is personally mediated racism, which includes assumptions made pertaining to intentions, abilities, and motives of an identified race.[12] The third is internalize racism, which refers to the acceptance of negative messages by the stigmatized race.

Children can develop significant stress from racial discrimination, which significantly affects their physical, mental, and behavioral health.[13] American Academy of Pediatrics (AAP) President Dr Sara "Sally" Goza, MD, FAAP, states that racism affects the health of children before they are born. The AAP states that racism harms children of all races and ethnicities, and recommends that conversations focused on discussing racism occur with children and adolescents of all races and ethnicities.[13]

MENTAL HEALTH

Screening for mental health concerns and referral for appropriate evaluation of mental health concerns is crucial to identify at-risk children and adolescents who may otherwise be overlooked.[4] Pediatric primary care providers have the opportunity to assess and provide appropriate intervention for pediatric mental health concerns. The well-child appointment provides an opportunity to discuss and assess mental health topics in a manner that is routine along with other anticipatory guidance topics.[14] Undertreated and untreated mental health disorders in childhood are linked with substance use disorders, physical comorbidities, and overall greater cost to the health care system when they are adults.[6] Integrating mental health services into primary care settings for pediatric patients could improve mental health aspects for many pediatric patients. Approximately 70% of children and teens, aged 18 years and younger, visit their primary care provider at least annually.[6] Assessing and addressing mental health concerns during primary care appointments is one way to increase access. In addition, patients and caregivers typically have an established rapport with their primary care providers, which fosters an atmosphere of trust when discussing mental health concerns.[6]

Screening and tracking the mental health of pediatric patients allows early diagnosis and treatment of mental health disorders.[5] Pediatricians are frequently the providers who perform the regular screening of pediatric patients in order to identify at-risk children and adolescents.[7] There are a variety of screening tools that have been validated for pediatric patients. **Figs. 1** and **2**, **Table 1** present common pediatric mental health screening tools.[15,16]

Blood pressure screening is also important in children. There was a need for revised guidelines in children and adolescents because the guidelines from 2004 did not provide sufficient information on ambulatory blood pressure monitoring, and included obese children in the normative data.[3] The updated AAP Clinical Practice Guidelines aim to simplify the identification and classification of hypertension in adolescents.[17] One difference between the recent AAP Clinical Practice Guidelines for blood pressure screening in children and adolescents and the previous Fourth Report is that the data in the Fourth Report included overweight and obese children and adolescents. The inclusion of these data may have underdiagnosed hypertension by skewing the results.[18] Overweight and obese youth are at higher risk for hypertension, with prevalence ranging from 3.8% to 24.8%.[19] The recent Clinical Practice Guidelines update differentiates the definition of hypertension between children and adolescents, using 13 years as the differentiating age. Definition of hypertension in children: greater than or equal to the 95th percentile for age, sex, and height on greater than or equal to

GAD-7

Over the <u>last 2 weeks</u>, how often have you been bothered by the following problems? *(Use "✔" to indicate your answer)*	Not at all	Several days	More than half the days	Nearly every day
1. Feeling nervous, anxious or on edge	0	1	2	3
2. Not being able to stop or control worrying	0	1	2	3
3. Worrying too much about different things	0	1	2	3
4. Trouble relaxing	0	1	2	3
5. Being so restless that it is hard to sit still	0	1	2	3
6. Becoming easily annoyed or irritable	0	1	2	3
7. Feeling afraid as if something awful might happen	0	1	2	3

(For office coding: Total Score T____ = ____ + ____ + ____)

Fig. 1. Generalized anxiety disorder (GAD-7) screening tool.

PATIENT HEALTH QUESTIONNAIRE-9 (PHQ-9)

Over the last 2 weeks, how often have you been bothered by any of the following problems? (Use "✔" to indicate your answer)	Not at all	Several days	More than half the days	Nearly every day
1. Little interest or pleasure in doing things	0	1	2	3
2. Feeling down, depressed, or hopeless	0	1	2	3
3. Trouble falling or staying asleep, or sleeping too much	0	1	2	3
4. Feeling tired or having little energy	0	1	2	3
5. Poor appetite or overeating	0	1	2	3
6. Feeling bad about yourself — or that you are a failure or have let yourself or your family down	0	1	2	3
7. Trouble concentrating on things, such as reading the newspaper or watching television	0	1	2	3
8. Moving or speaking so slowly that other people could have noticed? Or the opposite — being so fidgety or restless that you have been moving around a lot more than usual	0	1	2	3
9. Thoughts that you would be better off dead or of hurting yourself in some way	0	1	2	3

FOR OFFICE CODING ___0___ + _____ + _____ + _____

=Total Score: _____

If you checked off any problems, how difficult have these problems made it for you to do your work, take care of things at home, or get along with other people?

Not difficult at all	Somewhat difficult	Very difficult	Extremely difficult
⑤	⑤	⑤	⑤

PHQ-9 Scores and Proposed Treatment Actions *

PHQ-9 Score	Depression Severity	Proposed Treatment Actions
0 – 4	None-minimal	None
5 – 9	Mild	Watchful waiting; repeat PHQ-9 at follow-up
10 – 14	Moderate	Treatment plan, considering counseling, follow-up and/or pharmacotherapy
15 – 19	Moderately Severe	Active treatment with pharmacotherapy and/or psychotherapy
20 – 27	Severe	Immediate initiation of pharmacotherapy and, if severe impairment or poor response to therapy, expedited referral to a mental health specialist for psychotherapy and/or collaborative management

Fig. 2. Depression screening tool: Patient Health Questionnaire-9 (PHQ-9).

Table 1
Screen for Child Anxiety-related Disorders (SCARED) anxiety screening tool

Child Version - Page 1 of 2 (To be filled out by the CHILD)

Directions:
Below is a list of sentences that describe how people feel. Read each phrase and decide if it is "Not True or Hardly Ever True" or "Somewhat True or Sometimes True" or "Very True or Often True" for you. Then for each sentence, fill in one circle that corresponds to the response that seems to describe you *for the last 3 months.*

		0 Not True or Hardly Ever True	1 Somewhat True or Sometimes True	2 Very True or Often True
1.	When I feel frightened, it is hard for me to breathe	O	o	o
2.	I get headaches when I am at school	o	o	o
3.	I don't like to be with people I don't know well	o	o	o
4.	I get scared if I sleep away from home	o	o	o
5.	I worry about other people liking me	o	o	o
6.	When I get frightened, I feel like passing out	o	o	o
7.	I am nervous	o	o	o
8.	I follow my mother or father wherever they go	o	o	o
9.	People tell me that I look nervous	o	o	o
10.	I feel nervous with people I don't know well	o	o	o
11.	My I get stomachaches at school	o	o	o
12.	When I get frightened, I feel like I am going crazy	o	o	o
13.	I worry about sleeping alone	o	o	o
14.	I worry about being as good as other kids	o	o	o
15.	When I get frightened, I feel like things are not real	o	o	o
16.	I have nightmares about something bad happening to my parents	o	o	o
17.	I worry about going to school	o	o	o
18.	When I get frightened, my heart beats fast	o	o	o
19.	I get shaky	o	o	o
20.	I have nightmares about something bad happening to me	o	o	o

(continued on next page)

Table 1
(continued)

Child Version - Page 2 of 2 (To be filled out by the CHILD)

		0 *Not True or Hardly Ever True*	1 *Somewhat True or Sometimes True*	2 *Very True or Often True*
21.	I worry about things working out for me	o	o	o
22.	When I get frightened, I sweat a lot	o	o	o
23.	I am a worrier	o	o	o
24.	I get really frightened for no reason at all	o	o	o
25.	I am afraid to be alone in the house	o	o	o
26.	It is hard for me to talk with people I don't know well	o	o	o
27.	When I get frightened, I feel like I am choking	o	o	o
28.	People tell me that I worry too much	o	o	o
29.	I don't like to be away from my family	o	o	o
30.	I am afraid of having anxiety (or panic) attacks	o	o	o
31.	I worry that something bad might happen to my parents	o	o	o
32.	I feel shy with people I don't know well	o	o	o
33.	I worry about what is going to happen in the future	o	o	o
34.	When I get frightened, I feel like throwing up	o	o	o
35.	I worry about how well I do things	o	o	o
36.	I am scared to go to school	o	o	o
37.	I worry about things that have already happened	o	o	o
38.	When I get frightened, I feel dizzy	o	o	o
39.	I feel nervous when I am with other children or adults and I have to do something while they watch me (for example: read aloud, speak, play a game, play a sport)	o	o	o
40.	I feel nervous when I am going to parties, dances, or any place where there will be people that I don't know well	o	o	o

(continued on next page)

Table 1 **(continued)**			
41. I am shy	o	o	o

For children ages 8 to 11, it is recommended that the clinician explain all questions, or have the child answer the questionnaire sitting with an adult in case they have any questions.
Parent Version - Page 1 of 2 (To be filled out by the PARENT)

Directions:

Below is a list of statements that describe how people feel. Read each statement carefully and decide if it is "Not True or Hardly Ever True" or "Somewhat True or Sometimes True" or "Very True or Often True" for your child. Then for each statement, fill in one circle that corresponds to the response that seems to describe your child *for the last 3 months*. Please respond to all statements as well as you can, even if some do not seem to concern your child.

		0 Not True or Hardly Ever True	**1** Somewhat True or Sometimes True	**2** Very True or Often True
1.	When my child feels frightened, it is hard for him/her to breathe	o	o	o
2.	My child gets headaches when he/she is at school	o	o	o
3.	My child doesn't like to be with people he/she doesn't know well	o	o	o
4.	My child gets scared if he/she sleeps away from home	o	o	o
5.	My child worries about other people liking him/her	o	o	o
6.	When my child gets frightened, he/she feels like passing out	o	o	o
7.	My child is nervous	o	o	o
8.	My child follows me wherever I go	o	o	o
9.	People tell me that my child looks nervous	o	o	o
10.	My child feels nervous with people he/she doesn't know well	o	o	o
11.	My child gets stomachaches at school	o	o	o
12.	When my child gets frightened, he/she feels like he/she is going crazy	o	o	o
13.	My child worries about sleeping alone	o	o	o
14.	My child worries about being as good as other kids	o	o	o
15.	When he/she gets frightened, he/she feels like things are not real	o	o	o
16.	My child has nightmares about something bad happening to his/her parents	o	o	o
17.	My child worries about going to school	o	o	o
18.	When my child gets frightened, his/her heart beats fast	o	o	o
19.	He/she gets shaky	o	o	o

(continued on next page)

Table 1 (continued)			
20. My child has nightmares about something bad happening to him/her	o	o	o

Parent Version - Page 2 of 2 (To be filled out by the PARENT)

	0 Not True or Hardly Ever True	1 Somewhat True or Sometimes True	2 Very True or Often True
21. My child worries about things working out for him/her	o	o	o
22. When my child gets frightened, he/she sweats a lot	o	o	o
23. My child is a worrier	o	o	o
24. My child gets really frightened for no reason at all	o	o	o
25. My child is afraid to be alone in the house	o	o	o
26. It is hard for my child to talk with people he/she doesn't know well	o	o	o
27. When my child gets frightened, he/she feels like he/she is choking	o	o	o
28. People tell me that my child worries too much	o	o	o
29. My child doesn't like to be away from his/her family	o	o	o
30. My child is afraid of having anxiety (or panic) attacks	o	o	o
31. My child worries that something bad might happen to his/her parents	o	o	o
32. My child feels shy with people he/she doesn't know well	o	o	o
33. My child worries about what is going to happen in the future	o	o	o
34. When my child gets frightened, he/she feels like throwing up	o	o	o
35. My child worries about how well he/she does things	o	o	o
36. My child is scared to go to school	o	o	o
37. My child worries about things that have already happened	o	o	o
38. When my child gets frightened, he/she feels dizzy	o	o	o
39. My child feels nervous when he/she is with other children or adults and he/she has to do something while they watch him/her (for example: read aloud, speak, play a game, play a sport)	o	o	o
40. My child feels nervous when he/she is going to parties, dances, or any place where there will be people that he/she doesn't know well	o	o	o

(continued on next page)

Table 1
(continued)

| 41. | My child is shy | o | o | o |

SCARED Rating Scale Scoring Aide
Use with Parent and Child Versions

Question	Panic/ Somatic	Generalized Anxiety	Separation	Social	School Avoidance
1					
2					
3					
4					
5					
6					
7					
8					
9					
10					
11					
12					
13					
14					
15					
16					
17					
18					
19					
20					
21					
22					
23					
24					
25					
26					
27					
28					
29					
30					
31					
32					
33					
34					
35					
36					
37					
38					
39					
40					
41					
Total					
	Cutoff =7	Cutoff =9	Cutoff =5	Cutoff =8	Cutoff =3

Total anxiety ≥ 25

0 = not true or hardly true
1 = somewhat true or sometimes true
2 = very true or often true

SCORING

A total score of ≥ 25 may indicate the presence of an **Anxiety Disorder**. Scores higher than 30 are more specific.

A score of 7 for items 1, 6, 9, 12, 15, 18, 19, 22, 24, 27, 30, 34, 38 may indicate **Panic Disorder** or **Significant Somatic Symptoms**.

A score of 9 for items 5, 7, 14, 21, 23, 28, 33, 35, 37 may indicate **Generalized Anxiety Disorder**.

A score of 5 for items 4, 8, 13, 16, 20, 25, 29, 31 may indicate **Separation Anxiety Disorder**.

A score of 8 for items 3, 10, 26, 32, 39, 40, 41 may indicate **Social Anxiety Disorder**.

A score of 3 for items 2, 11, 17, 36 may indicate Significant **School Avoidance**.

Used with permission from Dr. Birmaher. Developed by Boris Birmaher, MD, Suneeta Khetarpal, MD, Marlane Cully, MEd, David Brent, MD, and Sandra McKenzie, PhD. Western Psychiatric Institute and Clinic, University of Pgh. (10/95). Email: birmaherb@msx.upmc.edu.

3 occasions for children less than 13 years of age. For adolescents greater than or equal to 13 years of age, 130/80 mm Hg is diagnostic of hypertension, regardless of age, sex, or height.[18] In addition, the new guidelines renamed the previously termed prehypertension to persistently increased blood pressure to specify blood pressure values that are in the 90th to 94th percentiles.[19] Revised AAP Clinical Practice Guidelines present an algorithm for blood pressure measurement based on whether the reading is in a normal percentile or not.[19] The algorithm assists primary care providers in determining appropriate evaluation and management of abnormal blood pressure. There are a variety of factors that affect management recommendations, including race and gender. More male pediatric patients have high blood pressure than their same-age female counterparts. In addition, African American and Hispanic adolescents have higher rates of increased blood pressure than same-age non-Hispanic white adolescents.[19]

Table 2 lists resources for mental health concerns for patients, families, and providers.

IMPACT OF RACISM ON MENTAL HEALTH

Racism has significant impact on children. Primary care providers should encourage discussion among family members regarding racism.[12] One way that parents can discuss racism with their children is to acknowledge that sometimes people are treated differently based on the color of their skins, or where they live. Parents may need to reflect on their own implicit biases in order to ensure they are positive role models for their children when they interact with people who are different from

Table 2
Mental health resources for patients, families, and providers

Topic	Source	Web Site
Biofeedback	Seattle Children's	https://www.seattlechildrens.org/clinics/biofeedback/patient-family-resources
Mental health app: game based, for all ages (free)	SuperBetter	https://www.superbetter.com/
Mental health app (free)	Smiling Mind	https://www.smilingmind.com.au/
Breathe, think, do with Sesame app for kids (free)	Public Broadcasting System	https://www.sesamestreet.org/apps/?_ga=2.109677637.1101931364.1605496885-993195212.1605496885
Mindfulness for teens	Dr Dzung Vo	https://www.Mindfulnessforteens.com
Suicide Screening Questions	National Institutes of Health	www.nimh.nih.gov/asq
Suicide Severity Rating Scale	Columbia Lighthouse Project	https://cssrs.columbia.edu/
Patient Safety Plan Template	Suicide Prevention Resource Center	www.sprc.org/resources-programs/patient-safety-plan-template
National Suicide Hotline	National Suicide Prevention Lifeline	1-800-273-TALK (8255); English 1-888-628-9454; Spanish www.suicidepreventionlifeline.org
Crisis Text Line	Crisis Text Line	Text HOME to 741741 www.crisistextline.org

them, and when they discuss people who are different from them.[13] The AAP published the 2019 statement *The Impact of Racism on Child and Adolescent Health*. In this statement the AAP urges pediatricians to counsel families on the impact that racism has on children and adolescents.[13] In addition, the statement provides recommendations for equitable policies at all levels of government in an attempt to reduce disparities and to create social justice.[13] Dr Sadiqa Kendia, MD, FAAP, and her husband, Dr Ibram Kendi, commented in the AAP News that they urge pediatricians to consider racism to be a diagnosis, because this allows primary care providers to present the idea of racism as something that can be healed.[20]

Dr Ibram Kendi is the founding director of the Center for Antiracist Research. Drs Kendi recommend that, in order to effectively combat racism within communities, a systematic approach is necessary. One strategy to develop and continue a systematic approach is to collect and analyze racial data from community health organizations.[20] This type of systematic approach produces a surveillance of racial data that can help to identify disparities and identify practices and policies that require revision.[20] Communities must encourage policy makers to address the crucial need for community-based mental health services for youth who had been receiving these services through the school.[21] In addition, telehealth mental health services should be considered as a possible alternative option when in-person therapy is unavailable; however, not all students have the technology required to engage in telehealth.[21] The US Department of Health and Human Services is allowing platforms that are not compliant with the Health Insurance Portability and Accountability Act (HIPAA) to be used during the pandemic to meet the needs of patients.[21] Non–HIPAA-compliant platforms, such as Apple's Facetime or Google's Duo, provide alternative options for virtual patient care. Although telehealth is a promising option, often children and adolescents are living in situations where there are multiple people in the home, and privacy may not be possible because of the living situation. The lack of privacy could affect the amount of information the student shares with the therapist/provider.[21]

Table 3 lists resources for patients, families, and providers regarding race issues.

BLOOD PRESSURE

It is important to identify children who have hypertension in order to minimize morbidity from cardiovascular disease as adults.[15] Primary hypertension is the main diagnosis for hypertensive children and adolescents evaluated in referral

Table 3		
Resources for patients, families, and providers regarding race issues		
Topic	Source	Web Site
Talking to children about racial bias	Healthy Children	https://www.healthychildren.org/English/healthy-living/emotional-wellness/Building-Resilience/Pages/Talking-to-Children-About-Racial-Bias.aspx
Books for younger children discussing race issues	Public Broadcasting System	https://www.pbs.org/parents/thrive/childrens-books-about-race-and-diversity
Books for older children discussion race issues	Chicago Public Library	https://chipublib.bibliocommons.com/list/share/204842963/1357692923?page=1

centers in the United States.[19] Children and adolescents who have primary hypertension tend to be older than 6 years of age, have a positive family history of hypertension, and are often overweight or obese.[19] Children and adolescents who have risk factors for primary hypertension do not typically need evaluation for a secondary cause of hypertension.[19] Children who do not have risk factors for primary hypertension should be evaluated for causes of secondary hypertension.[19]

Screening all pediatric patients annually, beginning at the age of 3 years, for high blood pressure is an important component of the well-child check.[19] Appropriate blood pressure cuff size is important when obtaining blood pressure.[19] The bladder of the cuff should encircle 80% to 100% of the arm, using a cuff with a width-to-arm circumference ration of 0.45 to 0.55.[19] **Table 4** lists best blood pressure measurement practices.[19]

A detailed history is an important component of the annual well-child check, as well as assessment for hypertension. Important aspects of the history pertaining to blood pressure are perinatal history, past medical history, nutritional history, activity history, and psychosocial history.[19] Important perinatal history questions include maternal hypertension, complications with pregnancy or delivery, gestational age, birth weight, and any perinatal medical issues.[19] Nutritional history includes sodium intake and typical foods and beverages ingested.[19] Past medical history includes diagnoses that are secondary causes of hypertension, such as neurofibromatosis, endocrine disorders, environmental exposures (lead, cadmium, mercury), renal and renovascular disorders, and cardiac disorders.[19]

During the annual well-child check office visit, it is important to obtain a full set of vitals, including calculated body mass index (BMI). Comparative percentiles should be reviewed based on the patient's age and gender.[19] There are a variety of physical examination findings that may be abnormal on physical examination. **Table 5** lists physical examination findings that may be observed in patients who have hypertension.

Table 4		
Best blood pressure measurement practices		
Patient Preparation	**Cuff Size**	**Clinical Pearls**
Child should be seated, with back support, and feet uncrossed on the floor or on a stool	Bladder length should be 80%–100% of the circumference of the arm	Inflate the cuff 20–30 mm Hg more than the point at which the radial pulse is no longer felt
Child should rest for a few minutes before the blood pressure reading	Width of the bladder should be at least 40% of the circumference of the arm	Deflate the cuff at 2–3 mm Hg/s
Take blood pressure in the right arm	—	Record the measurement to the nearest 2 mm Hg
Bell should be placed over the antecubital fossa	—	—

Data from FLynn JT, Kaelber DC, Baker-Smith CM, et al. Pediatrics. Clinical Practice Guideline for Screening and Management of High Blood Pressure in Children and Adolescents. http://doi.10.1542/peds.2017-1904.[19]

Table 5
Physical examination findings associated with hypertension

Organ System	Physical Examination Finding
General	Obesity High BMI
HEENT	Proptosis Retinal abnormalities
Cardiopulmonary	Apical heave Exertional dyspnea Palpitations Tachycardia
Gastrointestinal	Abdominal bruit
Integumentary	Acanthosis nigricans Diaphoresis Flushing Striae
Neurologic	Muscle weakness

Abbreviation: HEENT, head, eyes, ears, nose, and throat.
Data from FLynn JT, Kaelber DC, Baker-Smith CM, et al. Pediatrics. Clinical Practice Guideline for Screening and Management of High Blood Pressure in Children and Adolescents. http://doi.10.1542/peds.2017-1904.[19]

Table 6
Anticipatory guidance topics and corresponding online resources for healthy lifestyle

Topic	Organization	Web Site
Healthy living overview	Healthy Children	https://healthychildren.org/English/healthy-living/growing-healthy/Pages/default.aspx
Nutrition	Healthy Children	https://healthychildren.org/English/healthy-living/nutrition/Pages/default.aspx
Nutrition	Centers for Disease Control and Prevention	https://www.cdc.gov/healthyschools/bam/nutrition/nutrition-facts-label.htm
Nutrition	US Department of Agriculture	https://www.choosemyplate.gov/
Emotional wellness	Healthy Children	https://healthychildren.org/english/healthy-living/emotional-wellness/pages/default.aspx
Blood pressure	Centers for Disease Control and Prevention	https://www.cdc.gov/bloodpressure/youth.htm
Physical activity	Centers for Disease Control and Prevention	https://www.cdc.gov/physicalactivity/basics/children/what_counts.htm
Physical activity during pandemic	Centers for Disease Control and Prevention	https://www.cdc.gov/physicalactivity/how-to-be-physically-active-while-social-distancing.html
Physical activity	US Department of Health and Human Services	https://health.gov/sites/default/files/2019-09/Physical_Activity_Guidelines_2nd_edition.pdf
Healthy schools	Centers for Disease Control and Prevention	https://www.cdc.gov/healthyschools/vhs.htm
Healthy schools	Centers for Disease Control and Prevention	https://www.cdc.gov/healthyschools/vhs.htm

PATIENT ENGAGEMENT AND ANTICIPATORY GUIDANCE

Children and adolescents need to be included in their health management.[19] It is important for providers to explain what changes are occurring inside children's bodies, and to explain why healthy lifestyle choices are important and how healthy and unhealthy choices affect their bodies.[19] Children and adolescents must be encouraged to engage in conversations with the providers and caregivers to include the patients in their care. Children and adolescents desire to be active participants in their health care.[19] In certain patients, home blood pressure measurement may be helpful once a diagnosis of hypertension has been made, but it should not be used to diagnose hypertension.[19] In addition, there are not many at-home automatic blood pressure devices that are validated for pediatric use.[19] At present, there are not sufficient data in the pediatric literature to recommend that caregivers check the blood pressure of all children diagnosed with hypertension, and the frequency of home blood pressure monitoring has not been established in the pediatric population.[19] Patient and caregiver education is important and assists patients and caregivers with understanding their diagnoses and necessary lifestyle modifications in order to work toward making healthier choices in hopes of minimizing morbidity.[19] **Table 6** provides various anticipatory guidance topics for parents and caregivers and corresponding online resources for healthy lifestyle.

SUMMARY

Screening for mental health disorders and screening for hypertension are important in the primary care of pediatric patients. There are a variety of screening tools that primary care providers can use during well-child evaluations to screen for mental health issues. The revised AAP Clinical Practice Guidelines provide information for primary care providers to optimize the screening and management of pediatric hypertension. Universal implementation of screening for pediatric hypertension and pediatric mental health issues can identify children in need of further evaluation and management, and can improve long-term outcomes.

CLINICS CARE POINTS

- Pediatric mental health concerns have significantly increased over the past 10 years.[4]
- Approximately 20% of children in the United States between the ages of 3 and 17 years experience at least 1 form of mental health disorder, including attention-deficit/hyperactivity disorder, issues with behavior, and mood disorders.[6]
- Children who have mental health or behavioral disorders often continue to have mental health and behavioral disorders as adults.[7] Children and adolescents often do not receive appropriate assessment and treatment of mental health concerns, such as depression, anxiety, loneliness, social isolation, and suicide.[4]
- Racism affects mental health, and the AAP urges pediatricians to counsel families on the impact that racism has on children and adolescents.[13]
- It is important to identify children who have hypertension in order to minimize morbidity from cardiovascular disease as adults.[15]
- Screening all pediatric patients annually, beginning at the age of 3 years, for high blood pressure is an important component of the well-child check.[19]

REFERENCES

1. Gassman-Pines A, Ananat ED, Fitz-Henley J. Pediatrics. COVID-19 and Parent-Child Psychological Well-being. 2020. Available at: http://pediatrics.aappublications.org/content/146/4/e2020007294. Accessed September 9, 2020.
2. Al Kilbria GM, Swasey K, Sharmeen A, et al. Preventing Chronic disease. Estimated change in prevalence and Trends of childhood blood pressure levels in the United States after Application of the 2017 AAP guidelines. 2019. Available at: https://doi.org/10.5888/pcd16.180528. Accessed September 9, 2020.
3. Samuels J. Clinical Hypertension. New Guidelines for hypertension in children and adolescents. 2018. Available at: http://doi10.1111/jch.13285. Accessed September 9, 2020.
4. Biel MG, Tang MH, Zuckerman B. Pediatric Mental Health Care Must Be Family Mental Health Care. JAMA Pediatr 2020;174(6):519–20.
5. Boat TF, Kelleher KJ. Fostering Healthy Mental, Emotional, and Behavioral Development in Child Health Care. JAMA Pediatr 2020;174(8):745–6.
6. Yonek J, Lee CM, Harrison A, et al. Key Components of Effective Pediatric Integrated Mental Health Care Models. JAMA Pediatr 2020;174(5):487–98.
7. Perrin EC. Promotion of Mental Health as a Key Element of Pediatric Care. Am Med Assoc 2020;174(5):413–5.
8. Coller RJ, Webber S. Pediatrics. COVID-19 and the well-being of children and families. 2020. Available at: https://doi.org/10.1542/peds.2020-022079. Accessed October 14, 2020.
9. Golberstein E, Wen H, Miller BF. Coronavirus Disease 2019 (COVID-19) and Mental Health for Children and Adolescents. JAMA Pediatr 2020;174(9):819–20.
10. Goyal MK, Simpson JN, Boyle MD, et al. Pediatrics. Racial and/or ethnic and socioeconomic disparities of SARS-CoV-2 infection among children. 2020. Available at: http://pediatrics.aappublications.org/content/146/4/e202009951. Accessed October 14, 2020.
11. Kemp C. American Academy of Pediatrics. Discrimination associated with mental health woes in black teens. 2014. Available at: https://www.aappublications.org/node/35772.full.print. Accessed October 14,2020.
12. Wyckoff AS. American Academy of Pediatrics. Public health leader shares insights on racism's effects on health. 2016. Available at: https://www.aappublications.org/news/2016/03/25/Racism031616. Accessed September 9, 2020.
13. Jenco M. American Academy of Pediatrics. 'Dismantle racism at every level': AAP president. 2020. Available at: https://www.aappublications.org/news/2020/06/01/racism060120. Accessed October 14, 2020.
14. Smith JD, Cruden GH, Rojas LM, et al. Parenting Interventions in Pediatric Primary Care: A Systematic Review. Pediatrics 2020;146(1):e20193548.
15. Oregon Health & Science University. Screen for child anxiety related disorders (SCARED). 2019. Available at: https://www.ohsu.edu/sites/default/files/2019-06/SCARED-form-Parent-and-Child-version.pdf. Accessed October 14, 2020.
16. Spitzer RL, Williams JB, Kroenke K. Pfizer. Available at: https://www.phqscreeners.com/. Accessed October 14, 2020.
17. Khoury M, Khoury PR, Dolan KM, et al. Pediatrics. Clinical Implications of the revised AAP pediatric hypertension guidelines. 2018. Available at: http://doi.org/10.1542peds.2018-0245. Accessed September 9, 2020.
18. Batisky D. Screening for pediatric hypertension: How many readings are enough? Clin Hypertens 2019;21:1358–9.

19. Flynn JT, Kaelber DC, Baker-Smith CM, et al. Pediatrics. Clinical practice guideline for screening and management of high blood pressure in children and adolescents. 2017. Available at: http://doi.10.1542/peds.2017-1904. Accessed September 9, 2020.
20. Korioth T. American Academy of Pediatrics. Featured speaker Kendi to pediatricians: Consider racism 'a diagnosis'. 2020. Available at: https://www.aappublications.org/news/2020/10/06/nce2020kendi100620. Accessed October 14, 2020.
21. Du T, Fernandez C, Barshop R, et al. 2017 Pediatric Hypertension Guidelines Improve Prediction of Adult Cardiovascular Outcomes. Am Heart Assoc 2019; 73(6):1217–23.

Preventative Medicine for Older Adults

Gina L. Hogg, MSPAS, PA-C, GMPA, SCAPA, AAPA

KEYWORDS

- Geriatric preventative care • Choosing wisely • Age-friendly health care
- Medicare wellness visits • Comprehensive geriatric assessment
- Geriatric syndromes

KEY POINTS

- Geriatric patients are unlike any other population of patients because of the complexity of their care and lack of evidence-based guidelines for routine care in the elderly population.
- Using the Age-Friendly Health Systems 4Ms framework is recommended to help guide quality, meaningful care to older adults while honoring their care goals.
- The American Board of Internal Medicine has created a campaign, "Choosing Wisely," to help guide quality care supported by evidence, not duplicative of care already provided, and free from harm.
- Regular preventative medicine is important for older adults to address acute changes when they occur.
- Knowing what to screen for and when to stop screening in geriatric patients is important to avoid overtreatment.

INTRODUCTION

In medicine, US Preventive Services Task Force (USPTF) provides guidelines for evidence-based recommendations on clinical preventative services, including screenings, counseling services, and preventative medicine. These recommendations apply only to those patients who have no signs or symptoms of the specific disease or condition under evaluation. When considering these recommendations, they may not apply equally to older adults. In general, older adults are rarely part of randomized controlled trials (RCTs), which makes it difficult to apply recommendations from studies that do not target their generation, and recommendations may be based on indirect evidence.

There are 2 notable initiatives to help guide the management of preventative care in older adults. The American Board of Internal Medicine Foundation has developed the Choosing Wisely initiative to help increase dialogue between providers and patients

The author has nothing to disclose.
Internal Medicine and Geriatrics, Medical University of South Carolina, 135 Rutledge Avenue, MSC 591, Charleston, SC 29425, USA
E-mail address: anton@musc.edu

Physician Assist Clin 7 (2022) 77–87
https://doi.org/10.1016/j.cpha.2021.08.001
2405-7991/22/© 2021 Elsevier Inc. All rights reserved.
physicianassistant.theclinics.com

on avoiding unnecessary medical tests, treatments, and procedures. The mission of Choosing Wisely is to promote conversations between clinicians and patients to help choose care that is supported by evidence, not duplicative of other tests or procedures already received, free from harm, and truly necessary.[1] Although the Choosing Wisely campaign was not implemented strictly for older patients, it offers important topics of discussion for making decisions to help avoid treatment overuse and waste.

The John A. Hartford Foundation and the Institute for Healthcare Improvement in partnership with the American Hospital Association and the Catholic Health Association of the United States have developed the Age-Friendly Health Systems initiative. This initiative is designed to meet the challenge of providing evidence-based practice to the ever-growing number of older adults at every care interaction. The goal of the initiative is to spread the 4Ms framework (Mentation, Mobility, Medication, and What Matters) to 20% of US hospitals and medical practices by 2020, see **Fig. 1**. The aim of Age-Friendly Health Systems is to follow evidence-based practices, cause no harm, and align with What Matters to the older adult patient and their family caregivers.[2]

Mentation includes preventing, identifying, treating, and managing dementia, depression, and delirium across different settings of care. Addressing Mobility ensures that older adults move safely every day to maintain function and do What Matters. When Medication is necessary, age-friendly medications that do not interfere with Mentation, Mobility, or What Matters to the older adult across settings of care should be used. Last, each older adult should be asked What Matters to know and align care with the patient's specific health outcome goals and care preferences including, but not limited to, end-of-life care and across settings of care.[3]

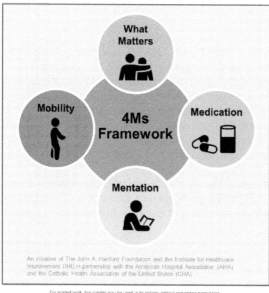

What Matters
Know and align care with each older adult's specific health outcome goals and care preferences including, but not limited to, end-of-life care, and across settings of care.

Medication
If medication is necessary, use Age-Friendly medication that does not interfere with What Matters to the older adult, Mobility, or Mentation across settings of care.

Mentation
Prevent, identify, treat, and manage dementia, depression, and delirium across settings of care.

Mobility
Ensure that older adults move safely every day in order to maintain function and do What Matters.

An initiative of The John A. Hartford Foundation and the Institute for Healthcare Improvement (IHI) in partnership with the American Hospital Association (AHA) and the Catholic Health Association of the United States (CHA).

For related work, this graphic may be used in its entirety without requesting permission. Graphic files and guidance at ihi.org/AgeFriendly

Fig. 1. Graphic developed by IHI to define the 4Ms of Age-Friendly healthcare. Reprinted from www.IHI.org/AgeFriendly with permission of the Institute for Healthcare Improvement, ©2021.

It is with these initiatives in mind that guidance is provided here for preventative medical care for older adults.

FACTORS TO CONSIDER IN OLDER PATIENTS

Geriatric patients have a variety of factors to consider as a patient population. As in any patient population, there are varying levels of high and low literacy, which can confound problems already existing due to hearing or vision impairment. Older adults are often not "tech savvy," which has made preventative and routine care visits difficult during this pandemic. Younger users may easily navigate a variety of platforms used for telehealth visits, whereas older adults often struggle to use these.

Functional impairment is another factor that leads to challenges. Older adults move more slowly and may have gait problems or sensory or cognitive deficits. These challenges all cause visits, whether in-office visits or via telehealth, to take a little more time and require a greater amount of patience.

According to the American Geriatrics Society (AGS), older adults should receive preventative health measures from which they are likely to benefit based on their health and remaining life expectancy using a person-centered approach and based on their clinical condition, which is broken down as

- Greater than 10 years of remaining life expectancy
- 5 to 10 years of remaining life expectancy
- Moderate dementia
- End of life

Preventative health recommendations for older adults need to be individualized based on health, function, risk of disease, and preferences, according to the AGS.[4] The purpose of screening is to identify cancers that will lead to poor outcomes if not found and treated early. Screening is not benign; patients may suffer anxiety, false reassurance from false-negative test results, complications from unneeded diagnostic evaluation (eg, bleeding from colonoscopy), and overdiagnosis, which leads to overtreatment. An example of this would be diagnosing and treating prostate cancer in an older male who may die of heart disease before prostate cancer.

MEDICARE WELLNESS VISITS

Patients who have had Medicare Part B for greater than 12 months qualify for an annual wellness visit to develop or update a personalized prevention plan to help prevent disease and disability, based on current health conditions and personal risk factors, along with a cognitive evaluation.[5] The wellness visit should include the following:

- Health risk assessment to help develop a personalized prevention plan
- Review of medical and family history
- Height, weight, blood pressure, and other routine measurements
- Review of current medications and health care providers
- Detection of cognitive impairment or frailty
- Personalized health advice
- A list of risk factors and treatment options
- A screening schedule for appropriate preventative services
- Advanced care planning

Unlike physical examinations or visits for acute conditions, the wellness visit allows the provider a chance to review the patient's current medications and health status and to determine what is working well for the patient. This is also an excellent opportunity to cover the 4Ms Framework with the patient and to document What Matters, current level of Mobility, check Mentation, and review Medication to determine if the patient may need some level of deprescribing.

Comprehensive Geriatric Health Assessment

Healthy lifestyle and nutrition

Living a healthy lifestyle at any age is important for longevity, and this is no different in older adults. Addressing healthy lifestyle choices at least once a year is important for maintaining the patient's health and safety. Patients should be counseled on smoking cessation, moderation with alcohol, diets rich in healthy fats, exercise, and strength training.

A diet rich in healthy fats that is low in transfats is associated with decreased overall mortality; Healthy Ageing: A Longitudinal Study in Europe (HALE) followed 70- to 90-year-old Europeans for 10 years and found that a combination of the Mediterranean diet, moderate to high levels of physical activity, moderate alcohol consumption, and nonsmoking status were associated with a 50% reduction in all-cause mortality.[6] Nutrition counseling referrals should be given for patient with a diet-related illness such as diabetes.[7]

Physical activity

Physical activity is important at all ages. In older adults, it helps prevent morbidity and mortality. Physical activity is also shown to promote functional independence, improve psychological health, and help prevents falls. Patients are recommended to get 150 minutes per week of moderate-level activity or 75 minutes of more intense activity plus muscle strengthening activities two times per week and balance strengthening activities 3 or more times per week in those at high risk for falls (AGS).

Tobacco and alcohol

At each visit, the patient should be asked about tobacco use, amount, and frequency and counseled on cessation. Both the US Surgeon General and the USPSTF recommend 3-minute counseling sessions with patients, with or without the use of medications, such as bupropion, varenicline, or nicotine products.[8,9]

Patients should also be screened for alcohol use at each visit to determine amount and frequency. In those patients who admit to alcohol use, the well-known CAGE (questionnaire that reliably diagnoses if a patient is drinking too much. C - Have you ever felt the need to cut down on your drinking? A - Have people annoyed you by criticizing your drinking? G - Have you ever felt guilty for your drinking? E - DO you need an eye-opener?) questionnaire has lower sensitivity in older adults. The AGS recommends the use of Alcohol Use Disorders Identification Test (AUDIT) or the Short Brief Michigan Alcoholism Screening Test-Geriatric Version (SMAST). Behavioral counseling may help those older adults displaying risky behavior and may also help reduce heavy drinking episodes. Counseling on alcohol use is important in older adults, particularly when they have mobility or frailty issues. Increased alcohol use contributes to falls, increased morbidity, and mortality.[4]

Aspirin for prevention

The use of aspirin as a prophylactic must be weighed carefully given that it puts the patient at increased risk of bleeding. USPSTF recommends the following:[10]

- Adults aged 50 to 59 years with 10% or greater 10-year cardiovascular disease (CVD) risk should take aspirin (unless at increased risk for gastrointestinal bleeding)
- In adults aged 60 to 69 years with 10% or greater 10-year CVD risk the decision should be individualized

Immunizations

- Older adults should receive their influenza shot annually. The intranasal influenza vaccine has not been approved for those older than 50 years.
- TDAP (tetanus diphtheria, acellular pertussis) should be given every 10 years.
- There are 2 types of vaccine for herpes zoster: Shingrix, which is given in 2 doses, 2 months apart, for adults older than 50 years, and Zostavax given in 1 dose for those older than 60 years.
- There are 2 pneumococcal vaccines, PCV 13 and PPSV 23. Adults older than 65 years who have not received PPSV 23 should first receive PCV 13, then PPSV 23 after 12 months.
- Adults older than 65 years who have received PPSV 23 should receive the PCV 13 1 year later.
- For adults older than 65 years who received PPSV 23 before the age of 65 years and will need to get a second dose, PPSV 23 should be administered 12 months after PCV 13 is given and at least 5 years after the most recent PPSV 23.[4]

Cancer Screenings

Prostate cancer screening

According to the American College of Surgeons, the benefits of prostate screenings, a modest reduction in morbidity and mortality from prostate cancer; the possible harms, over diagnosis/overtreatment; and the possible complications from treatment should be discussed when the patient is older than 50 years and has at least a 10-year life expectancy. The USPSTF recommendations are similar: discussing testing with patient aged 55 to 69 years with at least a 10-year life expectancy and recommends against testing in those older than 70 years.[11]

Breast cancer screening

According to the USPSTF, there are insufficient data on whether women should be screened for breast cancer after age 75 years. The Choosing Wisely campaign suggests not recommending breast cancer screenings to women with less than 10 years of remaining life expectancy. In patients with greater than 10 years of life expectancy, the pros and cons of mammography should be discussed every 2 years. There is no evidence that breast self-examination reduces morbidity or mortality.[4]

Colon cancer screening

The USPSTF recommends individualized plans for screening in those adults aged 76 to 85 years and does not recommend screening those older than 85 years because the risks do not outweigh the benefits.[4]

Lung cancer screening

The USPSTF has issued a draft recommendation statement, draft evidence review, and draft decision analysis on lung cancer screenings. Based on the review of evidence, the task force is recommending low-dose computed tomographic screening in adults aged 50 to 80 years who have a 20-pack per year smoking history and who currently smoke or have quit smoking in the past 15 years.[12]

Cardiovascular Screening

Blood pressure screening

The USPSTF recommends screening all adults for hypertension and confirming the diagnosis with blood pressure readings outside the clinical setting before starting treatment[13]; it recommends a home blood pressure monitor for the patient and have them keep a log to bring back to the next appointment. According to AGS,

15% to 30% of patients thought to be hypertensive have lower blood pressure outside the clinical setting[4]; this can often lead to patients being administered medication for hypertension they may not need.

Lipid screening

Low- or moderate-dose statin use has been associated with a reduced risk of all-cause mortality, cardiovascular mortality, ischemic stroke, and heart attack in an analysis of 19 RCTs of adults aged 40 to 75 year without CVD; however, very few trials include adults older than 75 years. In the 3 trials that included those older than 75 years (PROSPER, JUPITER, and HOPE-3), statins showed a moderate benefit for CVD but no overall change for mortality in those older than 75 years.[4]

- Screen for hyperlipidemia with a fasting lipid test.
- Starting statins for primary preventions should be a discussion with older adult patients. Patients should be aware of the risk for myopathy, possible increased risk of diabetes, and drug-drug interactions. The Mayo Clinic offers a decision maker at statindecisionaid.mayoclinic.org to help patients with making this decision.

Abdominal aortic aneurysm

The USPSTF recommends

- One-time screening of men aged 65 to 75 years who have ever smoked (defined as 100 or more cigarettes in lifetime) with a conventional abdominal duplex ultrasonography
- That clinicians selectively offer screening for abdominal aortic aneurysm (AAA) in men aged 65 to 75 years who have never smoked

At present, the USPSTF does not have sufficient evidence to conclude that screening in women aged 65 to 75 years who have ever smoked has any benefit and recommends against screening women aged 65 to 75 years who have never smoked. Medicare offers coverage of this screening for men and women with a family history of AAA only as part of the "Welcome to Medicare" preventative care.[14]

Diabetes

The American Diabetes Association (ADA) recommends that all adults aged 45 years or older be screened in the clinical setting every 1 to 3 years with a fasting plasma glucose, hemoglobin A_{1c} (HbA_{1c}), or oral glucose tolerance test. The diagnosis of diabetes is confirmed if there are 2 consecutive $HbA_{1c} > 6.5\%$, 2 consecutive fasting serum glucose greater than 126 mg/dL, or if both the HbA_{1c} and fasting glucose are greater their threshold.[15]

The ADA has a comprehensive set of guidelines for older adults because of concerns for overtreatment of diabetes, which can lead to hypoglycemia. The ADA recommends older adults be screened for cognitive impairment starting at age 65 years and yearly after that as appropriate.[16] Cognitive decline has been associated with an increase in inability to perform many self-care tasks, including taking medications appropriately. It is important to have a balance between appropriate glycemic control and preventing hypoglycemia.[15]

- The ADA recommends individualized medication plans for older adults.
- Older patients with few medical comorbidities and who are generally healthy with good cognitive function should aim for an HbA_{1c} greater than 7.5%.
- Older adults with cognitive impairment, coexisting chronic medical conditions, or functional dependence should aim for a relaxed goal of 8.0% to 8.5% A_{1c}.[15]

- HbA$_{1c}$ goals may be individualized to each patient's situation, but the overall goal should be to avoid acute hyperglycemia and hypoglycemia.

Comprehensive Geriatric Assessment

Assessing for geriatric health is an important part of the Medicare Wellness examinations. Comprehensive Geriatric Assessment (CGA) offers patients improvements in well-being, life satisfaction, continued performance of instrumental activities of daily living, and fewer clinic visits.[4] Elements of a good CGA include assessment of medications, cognitive status, functional status, nutritional status, hearing, vision, mental health, social support, gait, and balance (fall risk).

Cognitive assessment

According to the USPSTF, there is insufficient evidence to screen for dementia, whereas Medicare Annual Wellness Visits must include detection of cognitive impairment by direct observation with due consideration of concerns raised by the patient, family, or others.[5,17] Tests that may be used to assess cognition include

- Mini-Cog (clock drawing test combined with a 3-item recall test)[18]
- The Memory Impairment Screen[19]
- General Practitioner Assessment of Cognition[20]

Depression

Annual screening for depression is covered by Medicare. The USPSTF recommends screening adults for depression as long as the practice has the ability to treat and follow the patient.[21] The AGS recommends the following tools for screening:

- Geriatric Depression Scale[16]
- The one-question screen "Do you often feel sad or depressed?"
- Patient Health Questionnaire-2 ("Over the past 2 weeks, have you felt down, depressed, or hopeless?" and "Over the past 2 weeks, have you felt little interest or pleasure in doing things?")

Osteoporosis

- Routine screening (ie, measurement of bone mineral density through dual X-ray absorptiometry) is recommended by the USPSTF for all women aged 65 years or older and for women aged 60 years or older at high risk (as determined by the FRAX tool, www.shef.ac.uk/FRAX/) (AGS).[4,22]
- According to the USPSTF, evidence is insufficient to assess the balance of benefits and harms of screening for osteoporosis in men.[4]
- Screening men aged 65 years or older with a prior clinical fracture and all men aged 80 years or older has been shown to be cost-effective.[4]
- The National Osteoporosis Foundation recommends screening all men older than 70 years.[23]

Vision/hearing

There are no clear guidelines from USPSTF regarding hearing and vision screening in older adults.

- USPSTF found insufficient evidence for or against routine visual acuity screening by primary care providers. Clinical judgment should be used.[24]
- USPSTF also found insufficient data regarding routine screening for open angle glaucoma, although Medicare does cover this for those patients at risk.[25]

- USPSTF reports insufficient evidence to assess the benefits of routine hearing screens for hearing impairment.[26]
- It is important to note that screening for hearing impairment is a necessary part of the Medicare Annual Wellness Visit.
- According to AGS, pure tone audiometry is the gold standard for hearing assessment, but the whispered voice test at 2 ft has a 75% predictive value.[4]

Falls

Falls are the leading cause of injury in those older than 65 years and as such should be discussed at each visit.[4]

- Clinicians should ask patients annually about falls, balance, or gait problems.
- A multifactorial risk assessment for falls, which incorporates a focused medical history, physical examination, functional assessments, and review of extrinsic factors for older adults with 2 falls in the past year or 1 fall if combined with gait or balance problems assessed by a standardized gait and balance test.

Medication use

It is important at every visit to review medication use and to determine if patients are taking the medications as prescribed or if they have stopped any medications. Medications provide a wealth of tools for clinicians to help treat their patients' ailments. In discussing medication use, the practitioner can implement a discussion of the 4Ms framework. Discussing the medications that the patient is taking, any side effects, and any concerns they have about their medications can aid conversations about what the patient wants.

- Mentation: Is the medication causing any changes to cognition? Does the patient complain about how the medication makes them feel?
- Mobility: Is the medication contributing to changes in blood pressure, which causes them to fall, for example? Are they on sedating medications that affect mobility?
- Medication: Are the medications necessary for the life expectancy of the patient?
- What Matters: What does the patient want? Are they able to afford their medications? Are the medications contributing to their life in a positive or a negative way?

The concept of deprescribing has been promoted, and a guideline developed by the University of Montreal and the Bruyère Research Institute.[27] A mobile app has been developed to help aid practitioners in deprescribing medications for their patients.

Driving

There is not currently an effective, easily administered test to evaluate driving in older adults. The AGS does offer the Clinician's Guide to Assessing and Counseling Older Drivers (http://bit.ly/2FxUZw8) that may help the primary care provider in assessing their patients' fitness for continuing to drive. Otherwise, specific questions may be asked to help assess their ability to continue driving:[4]

- How did you get to this appointment today?
- Have you had any traffic violations, close calls, or accidents in the last 6 months? 1 year? 2 years?
- Have you gotten lost while driving?
- Do you feel comfortable continuing to drive?

Screening for elder mistreatment
The USPSTF does not show sufficient evidence for routine screening for elder abuse. Those patients who present with contusions, burns, bite marks, genital or rectal trauma, pressure ulcers, and body mass index 17.5 kg/m^2 or less with no medical explanation should be screened. These patients should be asked about abuse, and if necessary, referred to the local Department of Social Services.[4]

Screening for geriatric syndromes
The scope of this article has covered the individual screenings and recommendations in place for older adult patients. What is not specifically covered is the spectrum of geriatric syndromes. Major geriatric syndromes include frailty, cognitive impairment, delirium, urinary/fecal incontinence, dizziness, syncope, and depression. The term "geriatric syndrome" captures those clinical conditions that do not easily fit into specific disease categories, although the concept remains poorly defined.[28] Geriatric syndromes may seem distinctly different, but do share some common threads. These syndromes are very prevalent in older adults, especially frail older adults. Underlying factors and typically multiple organ systems contribute to and define geriatric syndromes.[28] Oftentimes, the patient's chief complaint will not necessarily relate to the pathologic process causing a change in health status. A common example of this is seen often in patients who present with delirium and are found to have a urinary tract or other infection present.

Geriatric syndromes are important to screen for because of their impact on quality of life. Recognizing these syndromes in primary care is vital to helping the patient move forward with the best quality of life they can, for as long as they can.

Frailty is an important component of geriatric syndromes and is defined by many as the "overarching geriatric syndrome" because it often may be a predictor of benefit and prognosis.[28] The most relevant clinical definition for the practicing clinician is a clinical syndrome including 3 or more of the following: unintentional weight loss, self-reported exhaustion, weakness, slow walking speed, and/or low physical activity. The frailty phenotype in elders followed over a 3-year period is independently predictive of incident falls, disability, hospitalization, and death.[29] In addition, older adults who were identified as frail were found to be at an increased risk of developing other geriatric syndromes.

SUMMARY

In conclusion, preventative medicine for older adults is multifaceted, requiring the practitioner to use evidence-based guidelines, clinical judgment, along with patient preferences to determine how to guide care for each patient. Although having enough time to spend with each patient can be difficult, spending the time to determine What Matters to the patient, evaluating Mentation, discussing Mobility, and determining if Medications are helping or harming the patient's goals is ideal to offer the patient goal-oriented care based on their wishes, recommendations, and their life expectancy. Additionally, familiarizing oneself with the Choosing Wisely campaign can help guide the patient toward choosing care that aligns with each individual's goals of care while avoiding the cost and risks of extraneous testing and/or procedures.

CLINICS CARE POINTS

- The Medicare Annual Wellness visit is a comprehensive annual visit that helps guide the care of geriatric patients.

- Geriatric patients are unlike any other patient population given they often have multiple comorbid conditions. Shared decision making between the provider, patient, and/or patient's family is ideal to meet the patient's needs for quality of life.
- Incorporating the 4Ms (Mentation, Mobility, Medications, and What Matters) and/or Choosing Wisely campaigns into the management of geriatric patients helps provide quality care without sacrificing the patient's wishes for their health care.
- Identifying geriatric syndromes in the geriatric patient impacts quality of life. Screening for and addressing the patient's needs as they become frailer ensures they maintain quality of life.

REFERENCES

1. Choosing Wisely. Available at: https://www.choosingwisely.org/our-mission/. Accessed December 5, 2020.
2. Age Friendly Health Systems. Available at: http://www.ihi.org/Engage/Initiatives/Age-Friendly-Health-Systems/Pages/default.aspx. Accessed December 5, 2020.
3. Age Friendly Health Systems. Available at: http://www.ihi.org/Engage/Initiatives/Age-Friendly-Health-Systems/Documents/AgeFriendly_4MsBySetting_Full Graphic.pdf. Accessed December 5, 2020.
4. Schonburg MD, Mars A, Sehgal MD, et al. Geriatrics review syllabus teaching slides. 10th edition. New York: American Geriatrics Society; 2019.
5. Medicare Yearly Wellness Visits. Available at: https://www.medicare.gov/coverage/yearly-wellness-visits. Accessed December 9, 2020.
6. Knoops KT, de Groot LC, Kromhout D, et al. Mediterranean diet, lifestyle factors, and 10-year mortality in elderly European men and women: the HALE project. JAMA 2004;292(12):1433–9.
7. U. S. Preventive Services Task Force. Behavioral counseling in primary care to promote a healthy diet: recommendations and rationale. Am J Prev Med 2003; 24(1):93–100.
8. U.S. Preventive Services Task Force. Counseling to prevent tobacco use and tobacco-caused disease: recommendation statement. Available at: http://www.ahrq.gov/clinic/3rduspstf/tobacccoun/tobcounrs.htm. Accessed January 5, 2021.
9. U.S. Department of Health and Human Services, Public Health Service. Treating tobacco use and dependence. 2000. http://www.surgeongeneral.gov/tobacco/treating_tobacco_use.pdf. Accessed January 5, 2021.
10. Aspirin Use to Prevent CVD and Colorectal Cancer: Preventative Medicine. Available at: https://www.uspreventiveservicestaskforce.org/uspstf/recommendation/aspirin-to-prevent-cardiovascular-disease-and-cancer. Accessed December 10, 2020.
11. American College of Physicians Releases New Prostate Cancer Screening Guidance Statement. Available at: https://www.acponline.org/acp-newsroom/american-college-of-physicians-releases-new-prostate-cancer-screening-guidance-statement. Accessed December 8, 2020.
12. USPSTF Recommends Lung Cancer Screening with Low Dose CT. Available at: https://www.aafp.org/news/health-of-the-public/20200715uspstfdraftlung.html#:%7E:text=Based%20on%20its%20review%20of,is%20a%20%22B%22%20recommendation. Accessed December 10, 2020.
13. Recommendation Statement on High Blood Pressure Screening in Adults. Available at: https://www.uspreventiveservicestaskforce.org/uspstf/document/RecommendationStatementFinal/high-blood-pressure-in-adults-screening#bootstrap-panel—3. Accessed December 10, 2020.

14. Abdominal Aortic Aneurysm: Screening. Available at: https://www.uspreventiveservicestaskforce.org/uspstf/recommendation/abdominal-aortic-aneurysm-screening. Accessed December 10, 2020.
15. Older Adults: Standard of Medical Care in Diabetes 2020. Available at: https://care.diabetesjournals.org/content/43/Supplement_1/S152. Accessed December 11, 2020.
16. Geriatric Depression Scale (short form). Available at: https://geriatrictoolkit.missouri.edu/cog/GDS_SHORT_FORM.PDF. Accessed December 11, 2020.
17. Cognitive Impairment in Older Adults. Available at: https://www.uspreventiveservicestaskforce.org/uspstf/recommendation/cognitive-impairment-in-older-adults-screening. Accessed December 11, 2020.
18. Standard Mini-Cog Instrument. Available at: https://mini-cog.com/mini-cog-instrument/administering-the-mini-cog/. Accessed December 12, 2020.
19. Memory Impairment Screen. Available at: https://www.alz.org/media/Documents/memory-impairment-screening-mis.pdf. Accessed December 12, 2020.
20. GPCOG Screening Test. Available at: https://www.alz.org/media/documents/gpcog-screening-test-english.pdf. Accessed December 12, 2020.
21. Depression in Adults Screening. Available at: https://www.uspreventiveservicestaskforce.org/uspstf/document/RecommendationStatementFinal/depression-in-adults-screening. Accessed December 28, 2020.
22. Osteoporosis to Prevent Fractures: Screening. Available at: https://www.uspreventiveservicestaskforce.org/uspstf/recommendation/osteoporosis-screening. Accessed December 28, 2020.
23. Clinical Guide to Prevention and Treatment of Osteoporosis. Available at: https://static1.squarespace.com/static/5d7aabc5368b54332c55df72/t/5d9f679cbc775a5f22c91b61/1570727839254/Cosman2014_Article_ClinicianSGuideToPreventionAnd.pdf. Accessed December 28, 2020.
24. Impaired Visual Acuity in Older Adults: Screening. Available at: https://www.uspreventiveservicestaskforce.org/uspstf/recommendation/impaired-visual-acuity-in-older-adults-screening. Accessed December 28, 2020.
25. Glaucoma: Screening. Available at: https://www.uspreventiveservicestaskforce.org/uspstf/recommendation/glaucoma-screening. Accessed December 29, 2020.
26. Hearing Loss in Older Adults: Screening. Available at: https://www.uspreventiveservicestaskforce.org/uspstf/recommendation/hearing-loss-in-older-adults-screening. Accessed December 29, 2020.
27. What is Deprescribing? Available at: https://deprescribing.org/what-is-deprescribing/. Accessed December 29, 2020.
28. Inouye SK, Studenski S, Tinetti ME, et al. Geriatric Syndromes: Clinical Research, and Policy Implications of a Core Geriatric Concept. J Am Geriatr Soc 2007;55(5):780–91.
29. Fried LP, Tangen CM, Walston J, et al. Frailty in older adults: evidence for a phenotype. J Gerontol A Biol Sci Med Sci 2001;56:M146–56.

Call to Action
Multidimensional PA Well-Being Strategies

Eve B. Hoover, DMSc, MS, PA-C, DFAAPA[a], Kari S. Bernard, PA-C, PhD[b],*

KEYWORDS

- Well-being • Stress • Burnout • Wellness • Mindfulness • Individual
- Organizational • System

KEY POINTS

- Clinician burnout has profound effects on provider well-being and impacts the effectiveness and safety of patient care.
- Positive psychology practices, such as mindfulness and gratitude, may provide the PA a foundation for healthy self-care and an awareness of the harmful effects of the negativity bias.
- PAs, as health care leaders, pave the way for wellness by identifying process areas that may cause an undue burden on health care providers, and encouraging psychological safety, open communication, and elimination of the mental health stigma.
- Aligning with national clinician wellness initiatives, PAs are encouraged to prioritize self-care alongside organizational and national interventions.

INTRODUCTION

The PA profession has grown significantly since its conception in 1965. With 148,560 certified PAs in 2020[1] and an occupational model that allows PAs to change specialties without additional training, the PA profession is highly regarded by workforce specialists as part of the solution to physician shortages.[2] In 2021, US News and World Report rated the PA profession as the #1 job in health care and the #1 job overall.[3] Most PAs in one national sample reported being satisfied with their lives in general and with work.[4] PAs are not, however, immune to professional burnout.

Burnout is defined by physical and emotional exhaustion, depersonalization, interpersonal disengagement, and a decreased sense of personal accomplishment.[5,6] Burnout negatively impacts clinicians and patients, with correlations to medical errors, job turnover, and decreased patient satisfaction.[4] In a study of PAs, Dyrbye and colleagues[7] found that 41.4% of respondents had symptoms of burnout and high-risk job characteristics were excessive work hours and specialties such as emergency

[a] Midwestern University PA Program, 19555 North 59th Avenue, Glendale, AZ 85308, USA;
[b] Orion Behavioral Health Network, Anchorage, AK, USA
* Corresponding author. 17025 Snowmobile Lane, Eagle River, AK 99577.
E-mail address: ehoove@midwestern.edu

Physician Assist Clin 7 (2022) 89–102
https://doi.org/10.1016/j.cpha.2021.08.002   physicianassistant.theclinics.com
2405-7991/22/© 2021 Elsevier Inc. All rights reserved.

medicine, pediatrics, internal medicine subspecialties, and surgery. Compared with other US workers, PAs are more likely to experience burnout.[7] Within this context, a focus on wellness in the PA profession is essential.

The purpose of this review is to outline approaches to PA wellness aligned with the Quadruple Aim, which incorporates clinician wellness alongside the existing aims of affordable, effective, and patient-centered care.[8] First, authors will appraise evidence-based personal practices that PAs may implement to support personal well-being. An examination of organization-level practices aimed at preserving and enhancing clinician wellness will follow. The review will conclude with a discussion of specific national clinician wellness initiatives.

INDIVIDUAL WELLNESS STRATEGIES

The health care workplace is characterized by high levels of stress. Stress can be a motivator, leading to efficient task completion and inspiring innovative patient care.[9] However, when workplace stress exceeds healthy levels, it can trigger maladaptive coping behaviors.[10] Exacerbating the problem, health care workers often focus on the needs of others at the expense of their own and may not recognize when professional demands are overwhelming their coping mechanisms.[11] Practices instituted at the individual level may provide PAs insight into this phenomenon and a reprieve from the influence of work stress on their personal health. Although there is no universally effective stress management approach, clinicians may benefit from a variety of tools that can be applied to the daily challenges of practicing medicine.

Positive Psychology

Rather than focus primary research efforts on illness, stress, and burnout, positive psychology is an evidence-based field that aims to flourish and promote well-being rather than solely reduce ill-being.[12] Researchers in the field of positive psychology explore aspects of life that make the journey worth living and create strategies to thrive rather than just survive.[13,14] The positive psychology aspects of mindfulness and gratitude have correlated with physical and emotional health benefits for patients. Positive psychology practitioners have integrated their concepts into the management of obesity, diabetes, the opioid crisis, and the epidemic of loneliness.[15] Positive psychology also supports health care providers by promoting beneficial behavior changes and increased work productivity.[12–15]

Mindfulness

Mindfulness is the awareness of one's own thoughts and feelings as they arise without placing judgment on these experiences.[16,17] Although used by the members of the military, primary and secondary schools, and Fortune 500 companies, this evidence-based practice has also been incorporated into medical education training programs, a variety of medical institutions for staff and clinicians, and patient care.[14,16,18–23] Mindfulness may help clinicians recognize sensations as they arise, both pleasant and unpleasant, and respond in a way that prioritizes both clinician and patient well-being.

Mindfulness brings to light the negative implications of harsh inner criticism common among dedicated health care providers. Becoming aware of internal dialogue in a nonjudgmental fashion may cultivate the development of self-compassion. Self-compassion encourages providers to treat themselves with the same respect and kindness that they show daily to patients. This wellness practice leads to the development of compassion satisfaction rather than compassion fatigue,[24] improves patient care, and protects against burnout.[25]

Mindfulness-based practices have also been shown to support connection, communication, clarity, and focus,[14] which may all counteract factors that contribute to burnout such as social isolation, loss of control and autonomy, and challenges with work-life integration.[7] Decentering, a skill associated with mindfulness, is focused on the objective observation of experiences.[26] When faced with challenges during patient care, clinicians can apply objective observation to create a brief pause before responding to a situation. This small space may encourage the awareness that not all thoughts represent truth, and that autopilot reactivity may not be the clinician's preferred response.[26] Increased awareness of moment-to-moment experiences, along with a decentered perspective, may lead to improved connection, sense of control over self and the situation, and efforts toward prioritizing wellness to support work-life balance.

Mindfulness-based training in the workplace may boost provider resilience. In a systematic review and meta-analysis of studies evaluating interventions aimed to prevent or reduce physician burnout, workplace mindfulness and stress management programs were effective at decreasing mild to moderate levels of emotional exhaustion and depersonalization.[27] In another systematic review and meta-analysis evaluating randomized controlled trials of burnout interventions, authors found that programs targeting physicians were associated with small but significant reductions in burnout, and these effects were strongest among more experienced physicians and physicians working in primary care settings.[28] Spinelli and colleagues[29] conducted a meta-analysis of randomized controlled trials of health care professionals and trainees and found that various types of mindfulness-based training correlated with meaningful improvements in several aspects of postintervention well-being, including anxiety, stress, and self-compassion.

PAs and other health care providers may feel overwhelmed by excessive workload and inability to balance personal and professional responsibilities.[7] Wellness tools may not be plausible if they require significant time and effort to incorporate, given already existing time constraints.[30] Although the prototypical Mindfulness-Based Stress Reduction course is taught over the course of 8 weeks, there are additional effective, condensed approaches to developing knowledge of wellness concepts.[31] Gilmartin and colleagues[32] conducted a systematic review of hospital-based studies in which mindfulness interventions lasting less than 4 hours were offered to health care providers. Researchers found that these brief training decreased stress, anxiety, and burnout, and improved mindfulness and resilience measures among participants. Several other studies have shown beneficial outcomes from shorter curriculum and brief, but consistent, practice.[33,34] Consistent practice has been found to support neuroplasticity, functional changes to the brain that support emotional regulation, and increased levels of well-being.[35] Brief moments of mindfulness and focus on the breath lasting only a few seconds can be incorporated using the "Pause, Breathe, Respond" technique. This concept, taught in the Mindfulness for Medical Professionals Course (https://mindfullifetoday.com/mindful-life-medicalcourse/), is used to encourage nonjudgmental recognition of sensations arising in a given moment, to support wellness, and to decrease the risk of burnout.

Gratitude Practices

Gratitude practice has been shown to support wellness, mood, sleep hygiene, and life satisfaction. Developing a gratitude habit may also make positive life events more visible.[36,37] Gratitude practice involves giving thanks, expanding happiness toward others, and becoming aware of simple, yet powerful, moment-to-moment positive (and often ignored) experiences.[36] Gratitude can take the form of recognizing simple things or a formal practice (**Box 1**). Intentionally cultivating gratitude and welcoming

Box 1	
Gratitude practices	
Informal practice:	Noting simple things to be grateful for each day:
	• A warm cup of coffee before work
	• Hallway laugh with a colleague
	• Thank you note from a patient
	• A day when the EHR doesn't crash
	• Comfortable bed after a busy day
Formal practice:	Three Good Things[30,37,38]
	• An evidence-based positive psychology exercise
	• Participants document 3 things each day that went well and their role in bringing about each thing.

positive emotions may invite a sense of ease and well-being even during an otherwise difficult day.[36,37]

A brief, easily accessible practice called Three Good Things (see **Box 1**) was incorporated by the Director of Patient Safety at Duke University to support the well-being of frontline staff.[37] Health care workers were invited to document 3 good things, no matter how small, that occurred over the course of the day before going to sleep each day. Although this activity was only 2 weeks long, there were substantial benefits that appeared to also be sustainable for up to 12 months following the intervention. Participants were found to have a decrease in depression and burnout, as well as improved work-life balance, strengthened relationships, and less conflict with colleagues.[37] Three Good Things is a powerful tool that may be used as an individual strategy, but can also be implemented into teams and organizations to promote a culture of wellness.

Recognizing the Negativity Bias

PAs are trained to detect abnormalities and find solutions to problems. In general, the human race has a negative bias that developed to sustain survival and safety. Hanson and Hanson[36] explain that human brains are like Velcro for negative experiences and Teflon for positive experiences. In other words, humans retain and fixate on negative memories more readily than positive memories. Health care providers may have countless numbers of uplifting, professionally and personally rewarding patient encounters throughout the day and far fewer difficult experiences. Yet clinicians may ruminate about the isolated challenging events. Rather than learn from difficult experiences, personal and professional growth may be less likely as the clinician's self-doubt and judgment increases, and joy for medicine decreases. Awareness of positive psychology tools may encourage the clinician to direct heightened attention to positive, rewarding, and enriching aspects of life (and medicine) rather than "getting stuck" on negative experiences, and as a result, support wellness and minimize the risk of burnout. Clinicians (and all members of the health care team) should be encouraged to recognize and celebrate successes, both large and small.[39]

Application of Individual Well-Being Strategies

As the health care workplace may trigger burnout, health care providers need to recognize the importance of self-care practices. **Box 2** lists multiple examples of how to incorporate individual wellness strategies such as breathing exercises, a wellness transition routine, journaling, and boundary setting into one's daily life. There are expansive wellness resources available to learn more about the incorporation of small, yet meaningful changes to promote self-care. **Box 3** provides the author's top 5

Box 2
Summary of individual wellness strategies

Foundation of self-care	Wellness begins with a strong foundation of self-care practices: • Eating a balanced diet[40] • Adhering to an exercise routine • Ensuring healthy sleep hygiene[39] • Spending time in nature[41] • Reducing exposure to media[40]
Breathing practices	Visit the following Web sites to find examples of breathing practices relevant to health care workers: • Mindfulness for Healthcare Workers During COVID: https://www.mindful.org/mindfulhome-mindfulness-for-healthcare-workers-during-covid/ • Compassion With Equanimity Practice for Caregivers: https://www.youtube.com/watch?v=EHvX7_ib-F0
Wellness transition routine	Incorporate one of the following activities at the transitions between work and home to separate occupational stress from personal life: • Mindful movement such as a walk or chair yoga practice • Mindful breathing or another breathing practice • Calming, joyful, or invigorating music • Reduced digital or technological exposure such as avoiding social media or setting the phone to silent or vibrate[42]
Journaling	Maintaining a written narrative and personal reflection has many utilities: • Assists health care providers with wellness, coping, empathy, and connection with patients[43,44]
Personal boundary setting	Knowing limitations protects personal and professional well-being: • Healthy personal boundaries may improve the quality of patient care delivered[45] • Communicating personal boundaries to other members of one's medical team may improve accountability[39]

Box 3
Fast track your way to well-being

Top 5 Recommended Individual Wellness Resources	1. Resilient: How to Grow an Unshakable Core of Calm, Strength and Happiness. By Rick Hanson and Forrest Hanson, published by Harmony Books in 2018 2. Attending: Medicine, Mindfulness, and Humanity. By Ronald Epstein, published by Scribner in 2017 3. Coronavirus disease 2019 (COVID-19) and beyond: micropractices for burnout prevention and emotional wellness. By David Fessell and Cary Cherniss, published in the Journal of the American College of Radiology, https://doi.org/10.1016/j.jacr.2020.03.013 4. Brief mindfulness practices for healthcare providers - a systematic literature review. By Heather Gilmartin et al, published in the American Journal of Medicine, https://doi.org/10.1016/j.amjmed.2017.05.041 5. Mindfulness for healthcare workers during COVID website: https://www.mindful.org/mindfulhome-mindfulness-for-healthcare-workers-during-covid/

recommended individual wellness resources focused on the topics of mindfulness, negativity bias, and burnout prevention.

ORGANIZATION LEVEL SOLUTIONS

Individual-level wellness practices fortify physical, mental, and emotional health, and enhance resilience. However, the demands of the health care workplace may overwhelm even the most resilient clinicians. Certain aspects of the contemporary health care environment, like increasing documentation requirements that decrease patient engagement and increase electronic health record time, have been linked to a higher likelihood of clinician burnout.[46] Modifying such workplace stressors are often outside of the control of individual clinicians. Meta-analyses comparing the effectiveness of individual-level interventions with those aimed at the health care workplace in reducing burnout found that organizational interventions were more effective and long-lasting.[27,28,47] Shanafelt and Noseworthy[48] warn against relying on interventions targeting clinicians, as these may imply that burnout is a failure on the part of the individual, and not the greater health care system. Ideally, practices adopted by individuals occur alongside meaningful organizational changes.[46,49]

Work Process Improvements

Addressing aspects of the work environment that accumulate to cause daily distress may lead to early positive returns in well-being change efforts. Assessments of workload, workflow, task delegation, and time allotment for patient care may identify process areas producing undue burden on health care providers.[50] PAs are often at the forefront of care delivery and may authoritatively speak to process and quality improvement.[51,52] It is therefore critical for PAs to participate in workplace assessments and associated measurements of well-being so their valuable perspectives and experiences may be factored into interventions.

Team-Level Interventions

Several interventions can be implemented at the team level to enhance clinician well-being. Allowing workers to maximize their contributions to health care team productivity has correlated with positive well-being. Clinicians who contribute to the fullest extent of their capabilities report higher levels of team culture and lower levels of emotional exhaustion.[53] In an assessment of joy in the health care workplace, Sinsky and colleagues[54] found that members of primary care teams within which medical assistants (MAs) and nurses took on increasing levels of patient care responsibility demonstrated higher job satisfaction. The concept of maximizing scope of practice has been seen in PA studies as well. Tetzlaff and colleagues[55] found that oncology PAs who spent a larger percentage of time doing nonpatient care tasks were at a 12-fold increase risk of burnout as compared with PAs who maximized their patient care responsibilities. In another PA job study, DePalma et al[56] found that opportunities to expand scope of practice and procedural skills were among the top job satisfiers for a sample of cardiology PAs. If PAs can practice at the top of their scope, it may enhance well-being.

Interventions aimed at instilling consistency within health care teams have demonstrated improved well-being. Willard-Grace et al[53] found that more time spent working with the same MA was associated with less provider emotional exhaustion. Gregory and colleagues[46] evaluated the utility of assigning teams of 2 providers and 3 MAs to jointly manage patient panels on perceptions of workload. Physician participants demonstrated significantly less emotional exhaustion at 3- and 6-months postintervention. PAs and physicians alike may capitalize on the stability of the physician-PA team, which may provide similar team-based benefits to well-being.[57]

Team culture can also influence team members' well-being. Team culture is the underlying attitude driving how team members communicate, participate, and support one another, and has been associated with lower levels of emotional exhaustion.[53] For PAs, the idea of team culture may manifest as mutual respect, open communication, and support shared with collaborating physicians. If respect and communication are absent, poor team culture may emerge and negatively influence the well-being of both PAs and physicians.

Leadership

The way health care professionals are managed has implications for their sense of well-being. Shanafelt and colleagues[58] demonstrated that increasing leadership ratings of physician supervisors predicted lower burnout and higher satisfaction levels for physician subordinates. Multiple PA well-being studies have concluded that the quality of the physician-PA relationship has similar implications for PA well-being. Burned out respondents in a study by Bell and colleagues[59] were more likely to leave a free text response indicating a negative relationship with their collaborating physician. Tetzlaff and colleagues[55] found that, for the oncology PAs in their study, perceptions of better physician leadership correlated with lower burnout. Boosting the leadership capacity of health care supervisors may boost the well-being of those on their team.

Organizational Climate

Organizational climate describes the written and unwritten rules that dictate behavior in an occupational setting.[60] Psychological safety is one hallmark of an organizational climate that supports clinician well-being.[49] A psychologically safe climate allows clinicians to process difficult clinical outcomes in a supportive environment. A clinical program that embodies this concept is Schwartz Center Rounds, in which health care team members come together to process patient outcomes (**Box 4**).[61] Providing opportunities to overcome work-related stress in a supportive group setting may instill a greater sense of safety in seeking help when emotional responses to patient outcomes overwhelm coping mechanisms.

Authenticity is another characteristic of organizational climate shown to preserve clinician well-being. Health care leaders may leverage a climate of authenticity as an intervention in settings characterized by high levels of emotional labor. Emotional labor develops when employees must suppress or transform emotional reactions during conflict into socially acceptable emotional displays.[62] Studies have demonstrated associations between emotional labor and burnout.[62,63] A climate of authenticity involves team members expressing authentic emotions to one another as a means of interrupting the association between emotional labor and burnout. A climate of

Box 4	
Schwartz rounds (https://www.theschwartzcenter.org/programs/schwartz-rounds/)	
Who	Interprofessional health care team members
What	Discuss real patient cases and share insight from multiple perspectives
When	After difficult patient outcomes
How	In a supportive group setting
Why	Normalize emotional reactions to challenging patient outcomes and enhance teamwork, communication, and quality of care.

authenticity can provide a reprieve from emotional labor, in that providers can express their true emotions to team members without fear of rejection, embarrassment, or punishment.[63] The physician-PA team may serve as a ready-made climate of authenticity for PAs and physicians to process emotional labor.

Chronic exposure to workplace stress may leave health care professionals vulnerable to a disproportionate burden of psychological distress when compared with the general US population.[64] Health care providers treating mental illness readily refer patients to specialized treatment yet may avoid seeking mental health care themselves over concerns of disclosing such care to regulatory agencies and health care delivery organizations.[49] The culture of silence related to mental illness among clinicians is prevalent in health care settings.[65] Destigmatizing help-seeking for burnout and its consequences is an essential step in reassuring clinicians, like PAs, that it is safe and encouraged to use organizational well-being resources. **Table 1** includes a summary of interventions that may be implemented targeting various aspects of the organization.

NATIONAL CLINICIAN WELL-BEING INITIATIVES

National well-being advocates are advancing sweeping changes to the health care system. In 2019, the National Academy of Medicine's (NAM's) Committee on Systems Approaches to Improve Patient Care by Supporting Clinician Well-being released a

Table 1
Summary of organizational interventions to enhance clinician well-being

Target	Interventions
Work process	The American Medical Association's *Steps Forward* Web site (https://edhub. ama-assn.org/steps-forward) includes several resources to improve health care work processes: • Ensure optimal provider panel sizes • Implement team documentation to decrease clerical burden • Integrate previsit planning for patient appointments
Teams	Supporting several aspects of teamwork may enhance clinician well-being: • Create consistent team infrastructure between providers and support staff (ie, nurses or medical assistants)[46,53] • Maximize team member scope of practice[54–56] • Train teams in communication, collaboration, and conflict management[53]
Leaders	Building leadership capacity may positively influence leaders and their direct reports[58]: • Offer training and coaching to organizational leaders • Conduct 360° leader evaluations and provide actionable feedback on leadership effectiveness • Recognize the influence of leadership responsibility on leader well-being • Encourage leaders to model self-care behaviors
Organizational Climate	Organizational climate may be leveraged to support individual and team-level well-being: • Align organizational mission and values with actions taken at the department, team, and individual levels[48] • Measure the well-being of organizational members and analyze alongside other indicators of success[48] • Promote psychological safety and a climate of authenticity with programs like Schwartz Center Rounds[61] • Provide anonymous reporting hotlines and confidential mental health services that can be accessed after hours[66]

Table 2
Key components of the well physician-California program[47]

Target of Interventions	Services
All physicians in California	• Online mental health self-assessment modules • A vetted network of experts in physician mental health • Developing education that will meet continuing medical education requirements for maintenance of certification
Physicians at risk for developing burnout	• Peer Support Program
Physicians with burnout	• Professional Coaching (Mild-Moderate Burnout) • One Week Retreat (Severe Burnout) focused on recovery

consensus report summarizing the body of research regarding health care professional well-being and setting forth a series of system-level recommendations.[65] These proposals ranged in scope from intentionally cultivating positive work and learning environments for health care professionals and trainees alike to reducing administrative burden and harnessing technology to generate solutions. The report also emphasized the need for clinician burnout recovery programs and the importance of reducing the help-seeking stigma so that clinicians will actually participate in such programs.

Prominent health care establishments have been advancing similar organizational strategies in the decade leading up to the NAM report. At the 2013 Society of General Internal Medicine annual meeting, clinicians from multiple institutions across the United States together presented 10 steps to prevent burnout.[67] Among them was the incorporation of a clinician well-being metric onto the organizational dashboard that drives many decisions made by health care executives. Four years later, Shanafelt and Noseworthy[48] published 9 Mayo Clinic initiatives to promote engagement and reduce burnout, such as leveraging leadership capacity, high-functioning teams, and organizational culture to influence positive well-being at work. In 2018, authors representing the American Medical Association published the Charter on Physician Well-being.[68] The charter included multiple levels of commitment for clinician well-being stakeholders, including society, organizations, and individuals.

Some states are heeding the call to action (**Table 2**). The Well Physician-California program supports California physicians with targeted interventions based on burnout

Box 5
Fast track your way to well-being

| Top 5 Recommended National Wellness Resources | 1. *Taking Action against Clinician Burnout: A Systems Approach to Professional Well-Being.* A 2019 consensus report published by the National Academy of Medicine, https://doi.org/10.17226/25521
2. American Medical Association Ed Hub *Steps Forward* website: https://edhub.ama-assn.org/steps-forward
3. Charter on physician well-being. By Larissa R. Thomas et al, published in the Journal of the American Medical Association, https://doi:10.1001/jama.2018.1331
4. Advancing physician well-being: a population health framework. By Mickey Trockel et al, published in the Mayo Clinic Proceedings, https://doi.org/10.1016/j.mayocp.2020.02.014
5. Preventing a parallel pandemic — a national strategy to protect clinicians' well-being. By Victor J. Dzau et al, published in the New England Journal of Medicine, https://doi:10.1056/NEJMp2011027 |

risk.[49] PAs share many of the burdens driving physician burnout and should be included in such initiatives. Ideally, other states will follow California's example but go one step further by folding PAs into these offerings. **Box 5** lists multiple critical national wellness strategies that PAs may advocate for within their local communities.

SUMMARY

PAs represent important frontline champions of sustainable change to the practice of medicine. Leaders from NAM, NAM's Action Collaborative on Clinician Well-being and Resilience, and the Association of American Medical Colleges, respectively, recently published a national call to action involving 5 high-priority actions to prevent a parallel pandemic of clinician mental illness.[66] In addition to continued funding of organizational wellness programs, they called for the incorporation of Chief Wellness Officers into COVID-19 command centers, federal tracking of clinician well-being, and anonymous clinician hotlines for personal and patient advocacy. Finally, they advised the allocation of federal funds for frontline clinician health similar to what was provided to first responders during the 9/11 terrorist attacks. Their undergirding message for health care organizations is to not abandon clinician well-being initiatives already underway, while also stretching to meet the additive needs that have arisen because of the COVID-19 pandemic. PAs may answer this call to action by sustaining and advancing clinician wellness priorities, while simultaneously being mindful of their own mental health.

CLINICS CARE POINTS

- Escalating levels of burnout highlight the importance of prioritizing clinician well-being
- Healthy, satisfied members of the health care team safely and more effectively deliver quality health care to patients and communities
- Evidence-based practices, such as mindfulness, have been linked to reduced stress, improved well-being, and a variety of other health benefits in clinicians and patients
- Organizational and national initiatives to prioritize wellness are more important than ever to promote a health care community of wellness

DISCLOSURE

E.B. Hoover has nothing to disclose. K.S. Bernard would like to list Bernard Wellness Initiative as a disclosure.

REFERENCES

1. National Commission on Certification of Physician Assistants. 2020 statistical profile of certified physician assistants annual report. 2020. Available at: https://www.nccpa.net/wp-content/uploads/2021/07/Statistical-Profile-of-Certified-PAs-2020.pdf. Accessed September 2, 2021.
2. Dunker A, Krofah E, Isasi F. The role of physician assistants in health care delivery. 2014. Available at: https://www.nga.org/wp-content/uploads/2020/08/1409TheRoleOfPhysicianAssistants.pdf.
3. Best Healthcare Jobs. US News and World Report website. 2021. Available at: https://money.usnews.com/careers/best-jobs/physician-assistant. Accessed September 2, 2021.

4. Coplan B, McCall TC, Smith N, et al. Burnout, job satisfaction, and stress levels of PAs. JAAPA 2018;31(9):42–6.
5. Copur MS. Burnout in oncology. Oncology 2019;33(11):687522.
6. Trockel M, Bohman B, Lesure E, et al. A brief instrument to assess both burnout and professional fulfillment in physicians: reliability and validity, including correlation with self-reported medical errors, in a sample of resident and practicing physicians. Acad Psychiatry 2018;42(1):11–24.
7. Dyrbye LN, West CP, Halasy M, et al. Burnout and satisfaction with work-life integration among PAs relative to other workers. JAAPA 2020;33(5):35–44.
8. Bodenheimer T, Sinsky C. From triple to quadruple aim: care of the patient requires care of the provider. Ann Fam Med 2014;12(6):573–6.
9. McGonigal K. How to make stress your friend. Edinburgh: TED Global 2013 talk; 2013.
10. Gross JJ, John OP. Individual differences in two emotion regulation processes: implications for affect, relationships, and well-being. J Pers Soc Psychol 2003; 85(2):348–62.
11. Mull CC, Thompson AD, Rappaport DI, et al. A call to restore your calling: self-care of the emergency physician in the face of life-changing stress-part 3 of 6: physician illness and impairment. Pediatr Emerg Care 2019;35(8):585–8.
12. Seligman MEP. Positive psychology: a personal history. Annu Rev Clin Psychol 2019;15:1–23.
13. Macaskill A. Review of positive psychology applications in clinical medical populations. Healthcare 2016;4(3):66.
14. Katyal S. Diagnosing happiness: lessons from positive psychology. J Am Coll Radiol 2018;15(7):1040–4.
15. Lianov LS, Fredrickson BL, Barron C, et al. Positive psychology in lifestyle medicine and health care: strategies for implementation. Am J Lifestyle Med 2019; 13(5):480–6.
16. Daya Z, Hearn JH. Mindfulness interventions in medical education: a systematic review of their impact on medical student stress, depression, fatigue and burnout. Med Teach 2018;40(2):146–53.
17. Orellana-Rios CL, Radbruch L, Kern M, et al. Mindfulness and compassion-oriented practices at work reduce distress and enhance self-care of palliative care teams: a mixed-method evaluation of an "on the job" program. BMC Palliat Care 2018;17(3):1–15.
18. Dobkin PL, Hutchinson TA. Teaching mindfulness in medical school: where are we now and where are we going? Med Educ 2013;47(8):768–79.
19. Epstein R. Attending: medicine, mindfulness, and humanity. 1st edition. New York: Scribner; 2017.
20. Carmody J, Baer RA. How long does a mindfulness-based stress reduction program need to be? A review of class contact hours and effect sizes for psychological distress. J Clin Psychol 2009;65(6):627–38.
21. Barnes N, Hattan P, Black DS, et al. An examination of mindfulness-based programs in us medical schools. Mindfulness 2017;8(2):489–94.
22. van der Riet P, Levett-Jones T, Aquino-Russell C. The effectiveness of mindfulness meditation for nurses and nursing students: an integrated literature review. Nurse Educ Today 2018;65:201–11.
23. Hoover EB, Butaney B, Stoehr JD. Exploring the effectiveness of mindfulness and decentering training in a physician assistant curriculum. J Physician Assist Educ 2020;31(1):19–22.

24. Neff KD, Knox MC, Long P, et al. Caring for others without losing yourself: an adaptation of the mindful self-compassion program for healthcare communities. J Clin Psychol 2020;76(9):1543–62.

25. Atkinson DM, Rodman JL, Thuras PD, et al. Examining burnout, depression, and self-compassion in veterans affairs mental health staff. J Altern Complement Med 2017;23(7):551–7.

26. Hayes-Skelton SA, Calloway A, Roemer L, et al. Decentering as a potential common mechanism across two therapies for generalized anxiety disorder. J Consult Clin Psychol 2015;83(2):395–404.

27. West CP, Dyrbye LN, Erwin PJ, et al. Interventions to prevent and reduce physician burnout: a systematic review and meta-analysis. Lancet Lond Engl 2016; 388(10057):2272–81.

28. Panagioti M, Panagopoulou E, Bower P, et al. Controlled interventions to reduce burnout in physicians: a systematic review and meta-analysis. JAMA Intern Med 2017;177(2):195–205.

29. Spinelli C, Wisener M, Khoury B. Mindfulness training for healthcare professionals and trainees: a meta-analysis of randomized controlled trials. J Psychosom Res 2019;120:29–38.

30. Fessell D, Cherniss C. Coronavirus disease 2019 (covid-19) and beyond: micro-practices for burnout prevention and emotional wellness. J Am Coll Radiol 2020; 17(6):746–8.

31. Regehr C, Glancy D, Pitts A, et al. Interventions to reduce the consequences of stress in physicians: a review and meta-analysis. J Nerv Ment Dis 2014;202(5): 353–9.

32. Gilmartin H, Goyal A, Hamati MC, et al. Brief mindfulness practices for healthcare providers - a systematic literature review. Am J Med 2017;130(10):1219.e1–17.

33. Phang CK, Mukhtar F, Ibrahim N, et al. Effects of a brief mindfulness-based intervention program for stress management among medical students: the Mindful-Gym randomized controlled study. Adv Health Sci Educ Theor Pract 2015; 20(5):1115–34.

34. Demarzo M, Montero-Marin J, Puebla-Guedea M, et al. Efficacy of 8- and 4-session mindfulness-based interventions in a non-clinical population: a controlled study. Front Psychol 2017;8:1343.

35. Heuschkel K, Kuypers KPC. Depression, mindfulness, and psilocybin: possible complementary effects of mindfulness meditation and psilocybin in the treatment of depression. a review. Front Psychiatry 2020;11.

36. Hanson R, Hanson F. Resilient: how to grow an unshakable core of calm, strength and happiness. New York: Harmony Books; 2018.

37. Roberts P. Three good things: build resilience and improve well-being. Am Nurse Today 2018;13(12):26–8.

38. Rippstein-Leuenberger K, Mauthner O, Bryan Sexton J, et al. A qualitative analysis of the three good things intervention in healthcare workers. BMJ Open 2017; 7(5):e015826.

39. Swift Yasgur B. Seven tips for managing healthcare teamwork during a pandemic. Gastroenterology Advisor; 2020. Available at: https://www.gastroenterologyadvisor.com/practice-management/seven-tips-for-managing-healthcare-teamwork-during-the-pandemic-expert-interview/. Accessed December 3, 2020.

40. Fullana MA, Hidalgo-Mazzei D, Vieta E, et al. Coping behaviors associated with decreased anxiety and depressive symptoms during the COVID-19 pandemic and lockdown. J Affect Disord 2020;275:80–1.

41. Bratman GN, Anderson CB, Berman MG, et al. Nature and mental health: an ecosystem service perspective. Sci Adv 2019;5(7):eaax0903.
42. Newport C. Digital minimalism: choosing a focused life in a noisy world. New York: Portfolio; 2019.
43. Bartos S. Self-achievement through creativity in critical care. Crit Care Nurs Clin North Am 2020;32(3):465–72.
44. Hester M, Ingalls NK, Hatzfeld JJ. Perceptions of ICU diary utility and feasibility in a combat ICU. Mil Med 2016;181(8):895–9.
45. Bernard K, McMoon M. Reading between the lines for a solution to burnout. JAAPA 2019;32(9):48–50.
46. Gregory ST, Menser T, Gregory BT. An organizational intervention to reduce physician burnout. J Healthc Manag 2018;63(5):338–52.
47. Ahola K, Toppinen-Tanner S, Seppänen J. Interventions to alleviate burnout symptoms and to support return to work among employees with burnout: systematic review and meta-analysis. Burn Res 2017;4:1–11.
48. Shanafelt TD, Noseworthy JH. Executive leadership and physician well-being: nine organizational strategies to promote engagement and reduce burnout. Mayo Clin Proc 2017;92(1):129–46.
49. Trockel M, Corcoran D, Minor L, et al. Advancing physician well-being: a population health framework. Mayo Clin Proc 2020;95(11):2350–5.
50. Linzer M, Poplau S, Grossman E, et al. A cluster randomized trial of interventions to improve work conditions and clinician burnout in primary care: results from the healthy work place (hwp) study. J Gen Intern Med 2015;30(8):1105–11.
51. Pagel JK. Sustaining hospital financial health: a role for physician assistant leadership. J Am Acad Physician Assist 2015;28(5):9–10.
52. Boucher NA, Mcmillen MA, Gould JS. Agents for change: nonphysician medical providers and health care quality. Perm J 2015;19(1):90–3.
53. Willard-Grace R, Hessler D, Rogers E, et al. Team structure and culture are associated with lower burnout in primary care. J Am Board Fam Med 2014;27(2):229–38.
54. Sinsky CA, Willard-Grace R, Schutzbank AM, et al. In search of joy in practice: a report of 23 high-functioning primary care practices. Ann Fam Med 2013;11(3):272–8.
55. Tetzlaff ED, Hylton HM, DeMora L, et al. National study of burnout and career satisfaction among physician assistants in oncology: implications for team-based care. J Oncol Pract 2017. https://doi.org/10.1200/JOP.2017.025544.
56. DePalma SM, Alexander JL, Matthews EP. Job satisfaction among physician assistants practicing cardiovascular medicine in the united states. Health Care Manag 2019;38(1):11–23.
57. Essary AC, Bernard KS, Coplan B, et al. Burnout and job and career satisfaction in the physician assistant profession: a review of the literature. NAM Perspect 2018. https://doi.org/10.31478/201812b.
58. Shanafelt TD, Gorringe G, Menaker R, et al. Impact of organizational leadership on physician burnout and satisfaction. Mayo Clin Proc 2015;90(4):432–40.
59. Bell RB, Davison M, Sefcik D. A first survey: measuring burnout in emergency medicine physician assistants. J Am Acad Physicians Assist 2002;15(3):40–9.
60. Dickson MW, Mitchelson JK. Organizational climate. In: Rogelberg SG, editor. Encylopedia of industrial and organizational psychology. Thousand Oaks: SAGE Publications; 2007. p. 546–8.

61. Walton M, Murray E, Christian MD. Mental health care for medical staff and affiliated healthcare workers during the COVID-19 pandemic. Eur Heart J Acute Cardiovasc Care 2020;9(3):241–7.
62. Bartram T, Casimir G, Djurkovic N, et al. Do perceived high performance work systems influence the relationship between emotional labour, burnout and intention to leave? A study of Australian nurses. J Adv Nurs 2012;68(7):1567–78.
63. Grandey A, Foo SC, Groth M, et al. Free to be you and me: a climate of authenticity alleviates burnout from emotional labor. J Occup Health Psychol 2012; 17(1):1–14.
64. Shanafelt TD, Boone S, Tan L, et al. Burnout and satisfaction with work-life balance among US physicians relative to the general US population. Arch Intern Med 2012;172(18):1377–85.
65. National Academies of Sciences, Engineering, and Medicine. Taking action against clinician burnout: a systems approach to professional well-being. The National Academies Press; 2019. https://doi.org/10.17226/25521.
66. Dzau VJ, Kirch D, Nasca T. Preventing a parallel pandemic — a national strategy to protect clinicians' well-being. N Engl J Med 2020;383(6):513–5.
67. Linzer M, Levine R, Meltzer D, et al. 10 bold steps to prevent burnout in general internal medicine. J Gen Intern Med 2014;29(1):18–20.
68. Thomas LR, Ripp JA, West CP. Charter on Physician Well-being. JAMA 2018; 319(15):1541–2.

Community Health

Healthy Communities
A Physician Assistant's Perspective

Lauren Richardson, MSM, PA-C[a], David T. Dubé, DHSc, MSc, PA-C[b],*

KEYWORDS

- Active transportation • Community health • Community education • Public activity
- Affordable housing • Exercise access • Nutrition • Social cohesion

KEY POINTS

- Communities that focus on public health can reduce inequality and reduce health disparities from race or ethnicity, social status, income, and any other issues discovered in this community.
- To make physical activity happen, the activities or programs should be geared toward the individual community; we cannot take a "one size fits all approach."
- Safe homes provide an environment for children and adults to thrive and reduce physical and mental stress, as elevated crime levels lead to increased mental and physical stress, especially in children and adults.
- To promote healthy communities, we need the support of government (federal/state), local business employers particularly, and most importantly community members for change to occur.
- Primary care providers form sustained relationships with patients in a community and having a primary care provider as a usual source of care leads to better health outcomes, lower health care costs, and fewer health disparities.

INTRODUCTION

A community's resources and infrastructure impact the health and disease of individual members, but attention to the health of the community as a whole elevates the entire community. Communities that focus on public health can reduce inequality and reduce health disparities from race or ethnicity, social status, income, and any other issues discovered in this community. The President's Council in 1993 offered the following as a working definition for sustainable communities: "healthy communities where natural and historic resources are preserved, jobs are available, sprawl

[a] South College, School of Physician Assistant Studies, Principal Faculty, 400 Goodys Ln, Knoxville, TN 37922, USA; [b] Physician Assistant Program, University of New England, 716 Stevens Avenue, Hersey Hall 317, Portland, ME 04103-2670, USA
* Corresponding author.
E-mail address: ddube5@une.edu

Physician Assist Clin 7 (2022) 103–116
https://doi.org/10.1016/j.cpha.2021.08.003
2405-7991/22/© 2021 Elsevier Inc. All rights reserved.
physicianassistant.theclinics.com

is contained, neighborhoods are secure, education is lifelong, transportation and health care are accessible, and all citizens have opportunities to improve the quality of their lives."[1] According to Healthy People 2030, the social determinants of health are separated into 5 domains: education access and quality, economic stability, neighborhood and built environment, health care access and quality, and social and community context.[2] Despite the knowledge of what makes a healthy community, many Americans still live in a community that is deficient in one or more of these areas.

As physician assistants, we are often the bridge between our patients and community services. As we work within a community, patients come to trust and respect our opinions and recommendations. This puts us in a unique position to affect not only our patients but the community as a whole. It becomes very important that we know how our community is doing to better serve our patients. For example, if you are treating patients in an area where access to clean water and healthy food are an issue, you will likely focus on access to clean water and healthy food versus just education about nutritional habits. Only by seeing and learning about the struggles our patients have are we able to treat the whole patient, not just their disease presentation. As members of our community, we should also focus on giving back to the community through participation in free or reduced-cost health services, community service, and helping to identify gaps in community resources.

This article provides information and resources about clean water, healthy food, importance of physical activity (PA), community safety, community education, social cohesion in a community, and health care access. This information can be used to educate your patients and yourself about why overall community health matters, and what elements serve to make a community healthy. These elements will become especially important as our communities work to heal from the after-effects of COVID-19. So many people have had to make sacrifices because of loss of financial resources that will have long-term health implications. Over the next several years, we will need to come together as a community to use medical resources and community resources wisely as we look toward the future.

PHYSICAL ACTIVITY AND HEALTHY FOOD

We are all aware of the physical and mental health benefits of routine PA. Despite this knowledge, before the year 2020, only 53.3% of adults engaged in aerobic activity, and the percentage of adults partaking in strengthening exercises was only a mere 23.2%.[3,4] Since 2020 and the emergence of COVID-19, individuals have had to decide safe and effective ways to maintain or start healthy activity. COVID has affected all aspects of our lives, most importantly our health. Besides the ever-present fears of illness and loss of life that many have been affected by COVID-19, is the loss of jobs/income (less money for health foods, vitamins, gym memberships), closed gyms/sports activities ceased or canceled, stores with less inventory of food, people remaining indoors, and worsening unhealthy habits such as increased use of alcohol, tobacco, legalized, and illicit drugs.[5] The strategies to combat COVID-19 have mitigated the present threat of illness, but in turn may have opened the door to long-term health consequences secondary to increased sedentary lifestyles, isolation-induced depression, poor food choice, and/or lack of food choices (**Fig. 1**).[6] Lifestyle alternatives, procedures, and plans will be desperately needed to correct the damage incurred by inactivity over the past year. PA and healthy food options are 2 areas requiring attention. As we have learned, a lack of activity without adjustment to caloric intake manifests in weight gain and associated health conditions (see **Fig. 1**).[7,8]

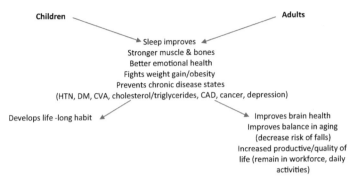

Fig. 1. Benefits of healthy activity among children and adults.[10]

Healthy Food

What we consume directly affects our well-being. Often, we are pressured by time, or the lack thereof, to consume unhealthy foods that are high in empty calories and sugar, as is the case with most soft drinks, which largely contribute to the increase in obesity levels across all ages.[9] The ability to obtain inexpensive food and drinks that are high in calories while providing no nutritional benefit, may be at the root of our current national obesity epidemic.[10] Not only has unhealthy food choices contributed to an increase in obesity, but sedentary lifestyles also compounded by restrictions on social interaction have caused the risk of obesity and cardiovascular disease to increase.[11,12] In a recent study, it has been reported that greater than 23% of the world's population is obese.[13] Not only is there a need to promote PA, but there is also a need to promote and provide strategies for healthy eating habits starting with school-aged children. This process can start with evaluation of daily/weekly caloric intake of community school breakfast/lunch programs. In addition, providing healthy food choices at reduced rates in vending machines within public-funded schools may be a good place to start.[14]

A much larger and concerning issue is the lack of or inability to obtain healthy foods. Many may find the concept of "food deserts" hard to believe, but in many communities, the presence of grocery stores or local corner markets is unmet.[15] In these communities, strategies need to be developed to combat the lack of healthy food alternatives. Measures have been taken in some regions to encourage local agriculture to partner with local businesses in an effort to improve access to healthy food options.[15,16] Some retail markets are providing space for locally grown foods and vegetables to be sold, which in turn promotes community well-being and pride.[16] Still, other communities support "farmers markets" whereby local community members bring to market excess fruit and vegetables, eliminating waste and instilling a sense of community caring and wellness.[17] On a larger scale, the federal government has recognized "food deserts," located predominantly in low-income areas, and has implemented policies and incentives to establish locations providing healthy food options.[18] In addition, federal and state government supported programs (SNAP/WIC) may allow for individual and family benefits to be used for the purpose of designated healthy food alternatives.[19]

Current strategies used in both the urban and rural settings strongly emphasize community gardening. The use of common areas, or green areas for the purpose of augmenting healthy food growth, has become widely acceptable. In urban communities, rooftop gardens have become widely accepted, providing healthy produce in areas often hardest hit by fresh produce shortages.[20,21] Community partnerships with local gardeners/farmers to use their expertise on-site selection to mitigate waste of resources, health hazards, and optimization of garden yield is essential to cooperative gardening as well as establishing gardening rules, roles, and responsibilities of community members.[22]

Physical Activity

As a result of health habit changes directly because of the fight against the COVID-19, health care and the communities in which they serve, need to partner in developing strategies to fight the surge of health conditions we may see in the very near future. Multiple studies have demonstrated that mixed land use is directly correlated with increased PA.[23,24] When people feel emotionally and physically safe in their communities, they are more likely to partake in active transportation such as walking or biking.[25] In addition, those individuals residing in well-designed communities where active modes of transportation are used to access shops, parks, and schools have demonstrated an overall increase in activity and lower body mass indices.[26] The development of communities, and revitalization of existing communities, should include plans to provide the opportunity to participate in safe PA. This may be paramount to mitigate the expected increase in demands on health care as a direct result of social distancing and isolationism.

The use of available resources to provide opportunities to walk or bicycle on designated areas of sidewalks and streets has been demonstrated to improve quality of life and well-being.[27,28] New communities should provide sidewalks to encourage walking, with existing communities updating community design through installation of safe, well-lit sidewalks with high visibility markings if they are not currently installed.[29,30] The promotion of cycling as a means of active transportation has demonstrated health benefits in a broad spectrum of ages. Bike lanes promote cycling and provide a level of needed safety benefits to users.[31] Community health benefits associated with biking can be leveraged through bicycling clubs where individuals socialize/exercise out of doors; and where applicable, bike to work with communities providing incentives to those who use this mode of transportation.[32]

The positive benefits of PA have been demonstrated, reducing health care costs to communities which promote development of health-minded communities.[30] Studies have shown when municipalities mandate construction of new planned communities to include playgrounds, sidewalks, stairs, and promote the use of green space, increased PA has been demonstrated.[33,34] Neighborhoods having access to parks or playgrounds within one mile of the community, exercise more than those individuals lacking access.[35] Thus, this emphasizes the need to incorporate multiuse space for play, social gatherings, and sporting events for individuals of all ages that are well-lit and safe. This should include the installation of water fountains and/or refilling hydration stations in all PA areas and not limited only to gymnasiums, but all parks, walking/cycling paths, playgrounds, or public areas which promote PA.[36,37]

How Do We "Make Physical Activity Happen?"

To make PA happen, the activities or programs should be geared toward the individual community; we cannot take a "one size fits all approach." Safety considerations regarding lower speed limits for residential areas with community activity spaces (bicyclists, skateboarders, walkers, children playing in streets) need consideration. In some locations, an increased presence of security guards or police regularly in public play/recreational green spaces may be all that is needed to promote use.

Community programs conducted year-round that use designated park or recreational land should provide those activities for adults and children of that individual community freely. The community may consider a "bring your own equipment" type program whereby participants share needed activity items and promote "no uniforms required" to keep costs low or no cost. Another strategy to encourage PA may be the development of new parks with adult equipment similar to, and alongside children's equipment. This will allow parents to exercise with, and at the same time as their children, instead of sitting, standing, or watching. Established parks could consider installing adult equipment to provide for family activities. These and many more ways to promote activity need the support of government (Federal/State), local business employers particularly, and most importantly community members for change to occur.

HOW SAFE IS YOUR COMMUNITY?

The overall safety of a community can have a significant positive or negative impact on overall community health. Some elements that contribute to the safety of a community are safe and affordable housing, crime rate, and childcare availability. Families who have safe and affordable housing do not have to make choices about paying for housing at the expense of nutritious food or even health care.[38] Safe homes provide an environment for children and adults to thrive and reduce physical and mental stress, as elevated crime levels lead to increased mental and physical stress, especially in children and adults.[39] Those who live in high crime communities are less likely to engage in PA or spend time outdoors, and children in increased crime neighborhoods are at an increased risk for depression, anxiety, and behavioral problems.[39] Childcare availability is important for early childhood development and for school-age children. Early childhood programs that focus on low-income families help to improve health access, provide early childhood education programs, and improve family outcomes.[40] After school programs provide social engagement, education support, and safety for many children.[41]

Safe and affordable housing continues to be an issue for many Americans. Over half of Americans report challenges with finding safe and affordable housing, and more than half of adults report making a trade-off when making housing choices such as taking a second job, moving to a less safe neighborhood, or sacrificing healthy food and health care to afford their rent or mortgage.[38] In many areas, the need for housing has outgrown the amount of housing available leaving families to make choices between housing, food, and health care.[38] The constant insecurity increases the mental and physical stress for both parents and children.[40] In addition, choosing cheaper low-quality food and not seeking preventative health care due to cost restraints lead to an increase in preventable conditions such as heart disease, diabetes, and obesity.

Crime in a community can also have a significant impact on health. Crime can be experienced through direct violence, witnessing of crimes or property damage, or hearing about crime that occurs in the community. People who are victims of violent crime or worry about becoming a victim may participate in less PA,[39] which leads to increases in obesity and other preventable diseases. Children who live in high crime neighborhoods are at risk for increased behavioral and mental health outcomes and exposure to violence can lead to an increase in aggressive behavior.[39] Crime reduction in low-income communities occurs through the availability of resources that provide for workplace development and improve access to affordable substance abuse treatment.[42] As the cost of college education has increased, many adults cannot afford workplace retraining, especially once they have already lost their primary income. Improved access and affordability of substance abuse treatment has long been known to have a significant impact on community crime, but while there is a disproportionately high amount of substance abuse in low-income communities, lack of access to treatment remains a significant barrier in most low-income communities.[42]

Early childhood development programs have been shown to have positive impacts on childhood mental and physical well-being as well as close education gaps. Programs such as Head Start focus on children from low-income households.[40] Not only do they provide childcare for working families, but also they focus on early childhood development and learning, providing nutritious meals, connecting families to health care, and supporting the well-being of families through programs that support parent-child relationships and involve the parents in childhood learning.[40] In addition to early childhood interventions, high-quality afterschool care has been shown to increase long-term earning potential, decrease crime and delinquency, and improve school performance.[41] These programs provide important social development opportunities, help with homework, PA opportunities, and safety for many youths.

COMMUNITY EDUCATION

Community-based education programs are an important part of a healthy community. Health education provides a strategy for implementing health promotion and disease prevention tailored to a target population. Health education can be presented on a large variety of topics such as smoking cessation, alcohol abuse, domestic violence, and importance of preventative health care. Many communities may also benefit from community subsidized workforce retraining programs. Identifying the needs of your community is the first step to developing a community-focused education program.

Early childhood and school-age educational programs should be implemented to teach early healthy habits. Nutritional education programs in addition to providing healthy school meals can build nutritional habits that last a lifetime helping to prevent or improve childhood obesity and diabetes rates in children. Programs in this age group should also focus on the dangers of smoking, alcohol, and drug use.[43] In middle school and high school-age children, additional programs should be presented that focus on pregnancy prevention and prevention of STDs including HIV and hepatitis C.[43] All age groups can benefit from education on the benefits of oral health, preventative health screenings, and importance of sunscreen use.[43]

Community-focused education programs that are targeted toward adults should provide support and education about smoking cessation, alcohol abuse, importance of PA, nutrition, and domestic violence. These programs need to focus on support to change habits as well as education on healthy habits. Many adults know what healthy habits they should practice, but due to circumstances such as lack of money or support, they struggle to implement those habits. Support groups for smoking cessation, alcohol abuse, or domestic violence provide a safe haven for discussion and support for change.[44]

Workforce retraining is lacking in funding and availability in most communities. When jobs leave an area, this leaves adults without resources to focus toward job retraining. Add in the rising cost of even a community college education, and many are forced to focus on having any job available to support their family at the expense of education that would allow them to increase their earning potential. Community subsidized education programs can help fill this gap and provide evening or weekend classes to working adults who wish to gain further vocational-based job training or pursue a college education.

Overall, attention should be given to the community needs and this can vary widely depending on the area of the country you live in. When working to increase community-based education, it is best to start with a community-wide evaluation to identify what opportunities are available to decide where to implement new programs. Many communities have resources that are just not well known and therefore not taken advantage of. It is important that as physician assistants we know what resources are available in our communities to point our patients in the right direction.

SOCIAL INVESTMENT IN COMMUNITY

A community's social investment can be seen through various channels. Strategies that promote community engagement, build social cohesion, and encourage philanthropy contribute to bolstering the health of a community.

Community Engagement

Community engagement is a core component of community health, and it occurs when a local community health system with community members and resources work together to plan, design, govern, and work to deliver health care services.[45] The WHO defines community engagement as, "a process of developing relationships that enable stakeholders to work together to address health-related issues and promote well-being to achieve positive health impact and outcomes."[45] Tamara Dubowitz and colleagues found that focusing on each individuals' sense of community and on activities that focus community health can be associated with improved community health, population health, and increased health civic engagement.[46] They collected 7187 nationally representative respondents from the 2018 National Survey of Health Attitudes and evaluated the associations between sense of community, community health investment, and barriers to investing in community health.[46] It was determined that individual engagement in the community may influence well-being for all.[46]

Social Cohesion

Healthy People 2030 separates the social determinants of health into 5 domains, one of which is Social and Community Context of Health.[47] "Social cohesion" is identified as the key issue in this domain. Social cohesion is defined as "the strength of the relationships and the sense of solidarity among members of a community."[48] Social cohesion can be further separated into 5 dimensions: social equality, social inclusion, social development, social capital, and social diversity.[49] Ying-Chih Chuang identified these through factor analysis and a multilevel analysis, which showed that participants living in countries with higher social inclusion, social capital, and social diversity were more likely to report good health that was not just a consequence of individual differences.[49]

Individuals use social networks to access the dimensions of social cohesion. These networks serve emotional, instrumental, or logistical support. Izet Masic defines social networks are structures made of individuals or organizations with one or more types of interdependent relationships such as jobs or friends that are used for exchanging information, knowledge, or financial assistance.[50] Social cohesion has benefits to residents of communities across all ages. Many studies support individual populations such as gender, diversity, and age all benefit from strong social networks. For example, Fan Wu and colleagues found that the influence of a family and friend network was weaker than that of a neighbor network on healthy aging.[51]

Authors of *Engaging Youth in Communities: A framework for promoting adolescent and community health* discuss the foundation of communities and identify the important roles communities play in shaping individual health using community-focused methods for understanding complex health issues and designing community-based solutions.[52] Parissa J Ballard, author of this study, proposes a fourth way.[52] She suggests thinking about the role of communities in individual health by proposing that "the community engagement process itself has implications for individual health and strong communities."[52] She notes that this is especially important during adolescence, as development during this time provides significant opportunities to instill the need to contribute to the world around us.[52]

Philanthropy

Most large employers participate in corporate philanthropy. Megan McHugh et al. conducted interviews with 13 of the largest US manufacturing companies to understand how these companies determined what cause to give money to and if the money was given to be focused improve a community's health.[53] Results indicated that giving was directed toward communities that had a large manufacturer presence, and while improving a community's health was not cited as a goal, funds were aligned with social determinants of health and not done in coordination with local public health agencies.[53] The authors contest there is an indication to better align public health and a community's corporate philanthropic goals.[53]

Robert Wood Johnson Foundation's: *Why Healthy Communities Matter to Business*, notes that when regional businesses and employers invest in the health and the economic vitality of the communities for which they live, there is a measurable benefit to the regional economy.[54] Across the country, many philanthropic organizations engage in helping improve population health and health of communities. The Federal Office of Rural Health Policy (FORHP) is one example of a national organization that works to create new approaches to connect with rural communities and use effective targeting of resources.[55] They are one of the groups in the Rural Health Public-Private Partnership that works on highlighting the innovative work foundations and trusts that are working in rural areas.[55]

The health of a community is partially successful because of the social investment it places in itself. Communities whose members and organizations engage in community efforts, support cohesion through social capital and networking, and offer funding, time, and attention through philanthropic efforts are better adept in elevating the health and welfare of members and the community.

ACCESS TO HEALTH CARE

About 1 in 10 people in the United States do not have health care insurance and therefore do not get the health care services that they need.[56] Those without insurance are not able to afford the health services that they need. In many areas, access to primary care is dwindling, leading many patients to only seek care for acute issues that could be prevented by regular care of chronic illnesses and preventative screenings.[56] In other areas, access to health care is limited by distance. Healthy People 2030 was launched during the middle of the COVID-19 pandemic with a vision of "a society in which all people can achieve their full potential for health and well-being across the lifespan."[57] Throughout the past year, the COVID-19 epidemic has highlighted the pervasiveness of health disparities. Many Americans fall into the high-risk category for COVID-19 because of underlying health conditions that are reflective of disparities in access to health care and underlying social determinants of health.[58] Health care disparities contribute to health disparities but the two are not interchangeable.[59] Health care disparities can many times represent inequalities in the process of providing health care to a community.[59] Disparities in health care quality that are persistent can be caused by issues surrounding race, ethnicity, and socioeconomic status.[59] Community health centers must identify the health disparities that are occurring in their local community and implement focused quality improvement strategies.[59]

Health insurance coverage is an important determinant of whether a patient has access to health care. Uninsured children and adults under the age of 65 years are much less likely to have a usual source of health care (ie, primary care) than those with insurance.[60] Timely access to appropriate ambulatory care allows for the prevention of illness, management of chronic conditions to avoid exacerbations or complications, and reduction in emergency room visits.[60] Primary care providers form sustained relationships with patients in a community and having a primary care provider as a usual source of care leads to better health outcomes, lower health care costs, and fewer health disparities.[61]

Access to health care is another problem that exists in many communities. In many rural or low-income areas, access to care can be limited. Many times, there is no access to specialist care and in many rural areas, access to primary care is limited as well. This leads many to seek care a significant distance away. The ability to travel or the cost incurred to travel leaves many patients lacking basic care. Patients then only present for "emergent" conditions that could have been prevented with regular preventative care.

SUMMARY

Physician assistants can impact their communities by helping their patients receive the necessary services that contribute to them leading healthier lives. Often, patients know what they are lacking but are unaware of where they can seek help to take advantage of resources in their community that are available to them. Identifying the deficiencies and disparities within a particular community is a good start in addressing the needs that exist.

Issues that communities may struggle with include access to clean water and healthy food, engaging in PA, living in a safe environment, accessing community education, experiencing social cohesion, and accessing health care. There are many elements within these issues that physician assistants can help their patients address, once health care providers know how their local community is helping its residents.

Focusing on correcting a community's particular needs requires knowledge of local infrastructure and resources available, while also realizing the effect COVID-19 has had on the lives of those in the community. The loss of income because of lack of employment, along with the associated social and physical isolation that has been exacerbated by COVID-19, resulted in significant lifestyle changes for many people. Many communities that were already lacking in areas that affect health, were exacerbated by the pandemic and may require even more community-wide engagement for the well-being of their public health as a whole.

Collaboration of federal and state government-assisted programs, along with partnering local businesses and philanthropy, can result in corrective measures that invest in and address health-related issues. If community members and organizations come together and embrace one another's strengths, they can make opportunities to expand access and resources for a healthy and sustained community. The benefits of which will be a better quality of life for residents, decreasing health care costs, and a more economically viable community.

FOR FURTHER INFORMATION

- https://health.gov/healthypeople
- https://youth.gov/youth-topics/afterschool-programs
- http://thefoodtrust.org/
- https://www.cdc.gov/physicalactivity/downloads/pa_state_indicator_report_2014.pdf
- https://www.cdc.gov/healthyliving/index.html

CLINICS CARE POINTS

- Personal and community safety can have a major impact on patient's well-being and mental health. It is important to check with your patients on a regular basis about their personal life, ability to eat well, exercise, access health care, and refer to resources as appropriate.
- Be aware of patient education resources available in the community. Promote and prominently display community education opportunities where all patients can see them during their visit.
- Educate your patients on nutrition. This is best accomplished through small regular interventions with stepwise goals to prevent frustration with large-scale changes.
- As community health care providers, physician assistants should routinely volunteer in community health care events and screens to promote healthy living activities.

ACKNOWLEDGMENTS

The authors would like to thank Heather Bidinger MMS, PA-C, DFAAPA at St. Catherine University for her contribution to this work.

DISCLOSURE

The authors have nothing to disclose.

REFERENCES

1. Clinton WJ. Executive order 12852. President's council on sustainable development. 1993. Available at: http://envirotext.eh.doe.gov/data/eos/clinton/19930629.html. Accessed March 26, 2021.
2. Social Determinants of Health. Healthy people 2030 website. Available at: https://health.gov/healthypeople/objectives-and-data/social-determinants-health. Accessed March 29, 2021.
3. Centers for Disease Control and Prevention. Exercise or physical activity. In: FastStats homepage – disability and risk factors. 2021. Available at: https://www.cdc.gov/nchs/fastats/exercise.htm. Accessed March 2,2021.
4. King DM, Jacobson SH. What is driving obesity? a review on the connections between obesity and motorized transportation. Curr Obes Rep 2017;6(1):3–9.
5. Congdon P. Obesity and urban environments. Int J Environ Res Public Health 2019;16(3):464.
6. Petrakis D, Margină D, Tsarouhas K, et al. Obesity - a risk factor for increased COVID-19 prevalence, severity and lethality (Review). Mol Med Rep 2020;22(1):9–19.

7. Sanchis-Gomar F, Lavie CJ, Mehra MR, et al. Obesity and outcomes in COVID-19: when an epidemic and pandemic collide. Mayo Clin Proc 2020;95(7): 1445–53.

8. Dwyer MJ, Pasini M, De Dominicis S, et al. Physical activity: benefits and challenges during the COVID-19 pandemic. Scand J Med Sci Sports 2020;30(7): 1291–4.

9. Tran D, Maiorana A, Ayer J, et al. Recommendations for exercise in adolescents and adults with congenital heart disease. Prog Cardiovasc Dis 2020;63(3): 350–66.

10. Imoisili OE, Park S, Lundeen EA, et al. Daily adolescent sugar-sweetened beverage intake is associated with select adolescent, not parent, attitudes about limiting sugary drink and junk food intake. Am J Health Promot 2020;34(1):76–82.

11. Pietrobelli A, Pecoraro L, Ferruzzi A, et al. Effects of COVID-19 lockdown on lifestyle behaviors in children with obesity living in verona, italy: a longitudinal study. Obesity (Silver Spring) 2020;28(8):1382–5.

12. Lavie CJ, Ozemek C, Carbone S, et al. Sedentary behavior, exercise, and cardiovascular health. Circ Res 2019;124(5):799–815.

13. Seidell JC, Halberstadt J. The global burden of obesity and the challenges of prevention. Ann Nutr Metab 2015;66(Suppl 2):7–12.

14. Micha R, Karageorgou D, Bakogianni I, et al. Effectiveness of school food environment policies on children's dietary behaviors: a systematic review and meta-analysis. PLoS One 2018;13(3):e0194555.

15. Ohri-Vachaspati P, DeWeese RS, Acciai F, et al. Healthy food access in low-income high-minority communities: a longitudinal assessment-2009-2017. Int J Environ Res Public Health 2019;16(13):2354.

16. Gregis A, Ghisalberti C, Sciascia S, et al. Community garden initiatives addressing health and well-being outcomes: a systematic review of infodemiology aspects, outcomes, and target populations. Int J Environ Res Public Health 2021; 18(4):1943.

17. Milliron BJ, Vitolins MZ, Gamble E, et al. Process evaluation of a community garden at an urban outpatient clinic. J Community Health 2017;42(4):639–48.

18. Testa A, Jackson DB. Food insecurity, food deserts, and waist-to-height ratio: variation by sex and race/ethnicity. J Community Health 2019;44(3):444–50.

19. Johnson MO, Cozart T, Isokpehi RD. Harnessing knowledge for improving access to fruits and vegetables at farmers markets: interactive data visualization to inform food security programs and policy. Health Promot Pract 2020;21(3): 390–400.

20. Litt JS, Soobader MJ, Turbin MS, et al. The influence of social involvement, neighborhood aesthetics, and community garden participation on fruit and vegetable consumption. Am J Public Health 2011;101(8):1466–73.

21. Malberg Dyg P, Christensen S, Peterson CJ. Community gardens and wellbeing amongst vulnerable populations: a thematic review. Health Promot Int 2020;35(4): 790–803.

22. Eggert LK, Blood-Siegfried J, Champagne M, et al. Coalition building for health: a community garden pilot project with apartment dwelling refugees. J Community Health Nurs 2015;32(3):141–50.

23. Slater SJ, Christiana RW, Gustat J. Recommendations for keeping parks and green space accessible for mental and physical health during COVID-19 and other pandemics. Prev Chronic Dis 2020;17:E59.

24. Lynch M, Spencer LH, Tudor Edwards R. A systematic review exploring the economic valuation of accessing and using green and blue spaces to improve public health. Int J Environ Res Public Health 2020;17(11):4142.

25. Lesser IA, Nienhuis CP. The Impact of COVID-19 on physical activity behavior and well-being of canadians. Int J Environ Res Public Health 2020;17(11):3899.

26. Leone L, Pesce C. From delivery to adoption of physical activity guidelines: realist synthesis. Int J Environ Res Public Health 2017;14(10):1193.

27. Morrey LB, Roberts WO, Wichser L. Exercise-related mental health problems and solutions during the COVID-19 pandemic. Curr Sports Med Rep 2020;19(6): 194–5.

28. Rahman ML, Moore A, Smith M, et al. A conceptual framework for modelling safe walking and cycling routes to high schools. Int J Environ Res Public Health 2020; 17(9):3318.

29. Child ST, Kaczynski AT, Fair ML, et al. 'We need a safe, walkable way to connect our sisters and brothers: a qualitative study of opportunities and challenges for neighborhood-based physical activity among residents of low-income African-American communities. Ethn Health 2019;24(4):353–64.

30. Gunn LD, Mavoa S, Boulangé C, et al. Designing healthy communities: creating evidence on metrics for built environment features associated with walkable neighbourhood activity centres. Int J Behav Nutr Phys Act 2017;14(1):164.

31. Pan X, Zhao L, Luo J, et al. Access to bike lanes and childhood obesity: A systematic review and meta-analysis. Obes Rev 2021;22(Suppl 1):e13042.

32. Gu J, Mohit B, Muennig PA. The cost-effectiveness of bike lanes in New York City. Inj Prev 2017;23(4):239–43.

33. Klompmaker JO, Hoek G, Bloemsma LD, et al. Green space definition affects associations of green space with overweight and physical activity. Environ Res 2018;160:531–40.

34. Kondo MC, Fluehr JM, McKeon T, et al. Urban green space and its impact on human health. Int J Environ Res Public Health 2018;15(3):445.

35. Cohen DA, Leuschner KJ. How can neighborhood parks be used to increase physical activity? Rand Health Q 2019;8(3):4.

36. Park S, Onufrak S, Wilking C, et al. Community-based policies and support for free drinking water access in outdoor areas and building standards in U.S. municipalities. Clin Nutr Res 2018;7(2):91–101.

37. Long MW, Gortmaker SL, Patel AI, et al. Public perception of quality and support for required access to drinking water in schools and parks. Am J Health Promot 2018;32(1):72–4.

38. The need for affordable housing. Habitat for humanity website. Available at: https://www.habitat.org/impact/need-for-affordable-housing. Accessed March 10, 2020.

39. Crime and violence. HealthPeople.gov website. Available at: https://www.healthypeople.gov/2020/topics-objectives/topic/social-determinants-health/interventions-resources/crime-and-violence. Accessed March 10, 2020.

40. Head start services. Office of head start website. Available at: https://www.acf.hhs.gov/ohs/about/head-start. Accessed March 10, 2020.

41. Benefits for youth, families, & communities. Youth.gov website. Available at: https://youth.gov/youth-topics/afterschool-programs/benefits-youth-families-and-communities. Accessed March 10, 2020.

42. Community organizations have important role in lowering crime rates. Brennan Center for Justice website. Available at: https://www.brennancenter.org/our-

work/analysis-opinion/community-organizations-have-important-role-lowering-crime-rates. Accessed March 10, 2020.

43. Educational and community-based programs. Healthypeople.gov website. Available at: https://www.healthypeople.gov/2020/topics-objectives/topic/educational-and-community-based-programs. Accessed March 14, 2020.

44. Social determinants of health. Healthypeople.gov website. Available at: https://www.healthypeople.gov/2020/topics-objectives/topic/social-determinants-of-health. Accessed March 14, 2020.

45. Cabore J, Kelly E. WHO Community engagement framework for quality, people-centred and resilient health services. WHO. 2017. Available at: https://apps.who.int/iris/bitstream/handle/10665/259280/WHO-HIS-SDS-2017.15-eng.pdf. Accessed March 26, 2021.

46. Dubowitz T, Nelson C, Weilant S, et al. Factors related to health civic engagement: results from the 2018 National Survey of Health Attitudes to understand progress towards a Culture of Health. BMC Public Health 2020;20(1). https://doi.org/10.1186/s12889-020-08507-w.

47. Social Determinants of Health. Health.Gov website. Available at: https://health.gov/healthypeople/objectives-and-data/social-determinants-health. Accessed March 29, 2021.

48. Kawachi I, Berkman L. Chapter 8: social cohesion, social capital, and health. In: Berkman LF, Kawachi I, editors. Social epidemiology. 1st edition. New York: Oxford University Press; 2000. p. 174–90.

49. Chuang YC, Chuang KY, Yang TH. Social cohesion matters in health. Int J Equity Health 2013;12(1):87.

50. Masic I, Sivic S, Toromanovic S. Social networks in improvement of health care. Mater Sociomed 2012;24(1):48–53.

51. Wu F, Sheng Y. Social support network, social support, self-efficacy, health-promoting behavior and healthy aging among older adults: a pathway analysis. Arch Gerontol Geriatr 2019;85:103934.

52. Ballard PJ, Syme SL. Engaging Youth in communities: a framework for promoting adolescent and community health. J Epidemiol Community Health 2015;70(2):202–6.

53. McHugh M, Farley D, Maechling CR, et al. Corporate philanthropy toward community health improvement in manufacturing communities. J Community Health 2017;43(3):560–5.

54. Why healthy communities matter to businesses. Robert Wood Johnson Foundation website. Available at: https://www.rwjf.org/en/library/research/2016/05/why-healthy-communities-matter-to-business.html. Accessed March 26, 2021.

55. Rural Health Philanthropy. Rural Health Information Hub website. Available at: https://www.ruralhealthinfo.org/philanthropy. Accessed March 19, 2021.

56. Health care access and quality. Health.Gov website. Available at: https://health.gov/healthypeople/objectives-and-data/browse-objectives/health-care-access-and-quality. Accessed March 29, 2021.

57. Healthy people 2030 framework. Health.Gov website. Available at: https://health.gov/healthypeople/about/healthy-people-2030-framework. Accessed March 29, 2021.

58. Giroir B. Healthy people 2030: a call to action to lead America to healthier lives. J Public Health Manag Pract. Available at: http://ovidsp.ovid.com/ovidweb.cgi?T=JS&PAGE=reference&D=ovftw&NEWS=N&AN=00124784-900000000-99210. Accessed March 29, 2021.

59. Fiscella K. Chapter 14: eliminating disparities in health care through quality improvement. In: Williams R, editor. Healthcare disparities at the crossroads with healthcare reform. Boston (MA): Springer; 2011. p. 231–67.
60. Health insurance and access to care. National Center for Health Statistics. NCHHS Fact sheet. 2018. Available at: https://www.cdc.gov/nchs/data/factsheets/factsheet_health_insurance_and_access_to_care.pdf. Accessed March 29, 2021.
61. Access to health services. Healthypeople.gov website. Available at: https://www.healthypeople.gov/2020/topics-objectives/topic/Access-to-Health-Services. Accessed March 29, 2021.

Sexual Health Preventive Services
Screenings, Vaccination, and Counseling

Aislinn E. Hopkins, MSPAS, PA-C[a],*, Emily B. Douglas, MSPAS, PA-C[a],
Megan S. Ady, MSPAS, PA-C[b]

KEYWORDS

- Sexual health • Screening • Prevention • STI • Intimate partner violence
- Counseling • Vaccination • Sex and gender minority

KEY POINTS

- Sexual health screening for STIs has various recommendations and should be reviewed for particular patient populations.
- Sexual health counseling should be provided to all men, women, and adolescents regardless of their sexual orientation or gender minority status
- Sexual health counseling includes STI and contraceptive counseling, intimate partner violence counseling, as well as counseling on sexual function
- Vaccinations are recommended for various populations of patients to protect against certain viruses that can be sexually transmitted including hepatitis A, hepatitis B, and human papillomavirus.

INTRODUCTION

Sexually transmitted infections (STIs) are of great concern for public health in the United States. STIs are often asymptomatic and can lead to numerous health complications, including reproductive health problems, fetal and perinatal health problems, cancer, and facilitation of the sexual transmission of human immunodeficiency virus (HIV) infections.[1] In 2018 the Centers for Disease Control and Prevention (CDC) reported approximately 26 million new STI infections that year—many of the infections are of young people aged 15 to 24 years.[2] Therefore, screening and using guideline recommendations are of utmost importance for reducing STI prevalence.

[a] Division of Physician Assistant Studies, College of Health Professions-Medical University of South Carolina, 151-B Rutledge Avenue, MSC 962, Charleston, SC 29425-9620, USA; [b] Division of Physician Assistant Studies, Murphy Deming College of Health Sciences-Mary Baldwin University, 100 Baldwin Boulevard, Fishersville, VA 22939, USA
* Corresponding author.
E-mail address: hopkinai@musc.edu

Physician Assist Clin 7 (2022) 117–125
https://doi.org/10.1016/j.cpha.2021.08.011
2405-7991/22/© 2021 Elsevier Inc. All rights reserved.

There are more than 35 organisms that can be transmitted by sexual activity. This section discusses 8 of the most common organisms and reviews recommendations from the US Preventive Service Task Force (USPSTF), the CDC, and many medical associations that recommend several preventative sexual health screening services. Of note, the most up-to-date recommendations only specify recommendations for women and men; however, screening is recommended and inclusive for all genders.[1–4]

DISCUSSION
Sexually Transmitted Infections

Chlamydia and gonorrhea are 2 common bacterial STIs that are often concomitant, thus typically screened together. Women who are 25 years and younger who are sexually active should be screened every year. Women who are pregnant should be screened during each pregnancy. Older women with risk factors for STIs, such as having unprotected sex (sex without a condom), a new partner, or multiple partners, should also be screened for chlamydia and gonorrhea.[2] Men who have sex with women, even if asymptomatic, should be screened if sexually active. Men who have sex with men should be screened once a year if sexually active.[2,5] There are also broad recommendations from CDC guidelines to screen for gonorrhea and chlamydia every 3 to 6 months if the patient has unprotected sex, has history of an STI or has a partner who has multiple partners, uses illicit drugs, or has a partner who engages in any of these behaviors.[6]

Human papillomavirus (HPV) is a virus with numerous strains that can cause genital condylomas and cervical cancer. The CDC highlights that HPV is considered the most common STI.[1] Although HPV is the most common STI among all genders, there are no standard screening recommendations for men, only for women. The screening recommended is a combination of cotesting or separate, which includes Papanicolaou test (cytology) and HPV testing. The cytology strictly looks for precancerous/cancerous cells of the cervix, whereas the HPV testing specifically looks for HPV strains in the cervical cells. HPV causes approximately 70% of cervical cancer; therefore, screening with Papanicolaou test and HPV strain testing is imperative.[7] Recommendations have changed in recent years for screening and decreasing unnecessary procedures such as colposcopy due to research noting that certain HPV strains have slow oncogenesis, approximately 10 to 20 years.[7] The screening should start for women aged 21 to 29 years, who should be screened every 3 years with cytology alone and HPV testing every 5 years. Women aged 30 to 65 years of age should be screened every five years with cytology plus HPV testing or every three years with cytology alone. Screening is not recommended for women younger than 21 years.[8] Women aged 65 years and older require no screening if a series of initial tests were normal and they are not at high risk for cervical cancer.[2,5] There are no current approved screening recommendations for men for HPV testing. There are anal Papanicolaou tests, and they can be offered to men at increased risk for anal cancer, including men with HIV or men who receive anal sex.[9] However, the testing is up to provider discretion.

Hepatitis B is a virus that causes liver disease that can lead to acute or chronic disease processes with various complications; there is a preventive vaccine but no current cure, although hepatitis B can be controlled with treatment.[1,5] The spectrum of the varying disease process includes risk of end-stage liver disease, cancer, and viral load increasing risk for infecting others; therefore, screening is critical for assessing the condition and its progression.[10] Screening recommendations are for women who are pregnant; for men, women, and those who are at increased risk (at-risk individuals include patients who have had unprotected sex, have a history of an STI or a partner who has a history of STI, have multiple partners, use illicit drugs, or have a partner who engages in any of these behaviors[6]); as well as in HIV+ individuals.[1,5]

Hepatitis C is a virus that causes liver disease that can lead to acute or chronic disease processes, with various complications. Hepatitis C has no current vaccine or pre-exposure or postexposure prophylaxis; therefore, screening is vital.[11] Screening recommendations are for women who are pregnant; for men, women, and those who are at increased risk (at-risk individuals include patients who have had unprotected sex, have a history of an STI or a partner who has a history of STI, have multiple partners, use illicit drugs, or have a partner who engages in any of these behaviors[6]); as well as in HIV+ individuals.[1,5]

Syphilis is a bacterial infection with 3 stages and may go unnoticed; however, most damage is irreversible once at the tertiary stage, affecting neurologic, cardiovascular, and other organ systems. The CDC published a "call to action" document in 2017 noting the increased incidence of syphilis in the United States; therefore, screening is of utmost importance.[12] Screening recommendations are for women who are pregnant; for men, women, and those who are at increased risk (at-risk individuals include patients who have had unprotected sex, have a history of an STI or a partner who has a history of STI, have multiple partners, use illicit drugs, or have a partner who engages in any of these behaviors[6]); as well as in HIV+ individuals.[1,5]

Herpes simplex virus (HSV1 and HSV2) is a virus that can cause oral or genital herpetic lesions. There is neither a vaccine nor a cure for HSV. HSV screening recommendations are based on clinical history. Routine screening of asymptomatic patients is not recommended.[1,5]

HIV is a virus that weakens the immune system making the infected person susceptible to infections and currently has no effective cure. Screening recommendations are for women who are pregnant; for men, women, and those who are at increased risk (at-risk individuals include patients who have had unprotected sex, have a history of an STI or a partner who has a history of STI, have multiple partners, use illicit drugs, or have a partner who engages in any of these behaviors[6]) (test annually); and for those who are or have been sexually active (test at least once).[1,2,5,13,14]

Sexual Health Vaccinations

Vaccinations can prevent many diseases in our lives, including some that are transmitted through sexual activity. Currently, there are vaccinations to protect against diseases such as hepatitis A, hepatitis B, and cervical cancers caused by certain strains of the HPV. Although these vaccines may have recommendations for other patient populations or other purposes, this article focuses on the aspects that affect sexual health.[15–17]

Hepatitis A is a virus that is transmitted through fecal-oral contact.[18] Persons who engage in oral-anal sex are at a high risk of contracting hepatitis A. The CDC has recommendations for the hepatitis A vaccination for persons who engage in oral-anal sexual activity and men who have sex with men.[18] The hepatitis A vaccination is a 2-shot series that is given 6 months apart. Studies have deemed the hepatitis A vaccination safe and effective at providing long-term immunity after vaccination is completed.[16]

Hepatitis B is a virus transmitted through body fluids (blood, semen, and vaginal secretions) and can therefore be transmitted through sexual contacts.[19] Hepatitis B can cause any number of symptoms from mild illness to chronic infections affecting the liver such as cirrhosis and even more serious conditions such as liver cancer.[17] The CDC has recommendations for hepatitis B vaccinations for sexually active persons, those treated for STIs, men who have sex with men, and anyone who is sexually involved with someone who has a known hepatitis B infection.[19] The hepatitis B vaccination is a 3- or 4-shot series that is given over 6 months. Studies have deemed the hepatitis B vaccination safe and effective at providing long-term immunity after vaccination is complete.

HPV is a group of more than 100 viruses that infect bodily tissue.[15] Certain strains of HPV can cause warts on hands, feet, or genitals. Certain types of genital warts and strains of HPV can lead to changes of cells that live on a female's cervix and ultimately result in cervical cancer.[15] The HPV vaccine can help protect against certain types of HPV that are linked to causing cervical cancer. The CDC has recommendations for HPV vaccinations for all boys and girls starting at age 9 years.[20] The vaccine produces a more robust immune response in those who take it at an earlier age; it is given before becoming sexually active. Recommendations are in place that persons may receive the vaccine up to age 26 years. However, adults up to age 45 years may receive the offer to take the vaccine after their sexual history is known to their health care provider. For persons up to age 14 years, the HPV vaccine is a 2-dose series given over 6 to 12 months. For persons older than 14 years, the recommendation is then a 3-dose series that is delivered over 6 months. Studies have deemed the HPV vaccination safe. Overall, HPV infections and cervical cancers linked to HPV rates have dropped significantly, having vaccination recommendations in place, and herd immunity is being established.[1,15,21] Of note, among teenaged girls, HPV cases and HPV-linked cervical cancer occurrences have dropped 86%.[15] In young adult women, occurrences have dropped 71%.[15]

Sexual Health Counseling

Comprehensive sexual preventative care includes counseling based on personal risk factors and patient age. Once risk factors are identified via screening (STI risk, depression, anxiety, substance use, etc.), counseling can further understand health risk and risk management. Several counseling points should be discussed with every patient at their preventive medicine visit. However, clinician judgment should be used to determine which patients to counsel.

Intimate partner violence

Intimate partner violence (IPV) should be screened for in all adolescents and women annually.[22] If risk factors or history of IPV are identified, the provider should provide education, referral for appropriate services, and referral for counseling.[22] Clinicians should ask questions regarding IPV in a private and confidential setting, and patients should be separated from partners before screening. The provider should also consider the increased risk of IPV experienced within the sex and gender minority community and include inclusive screening for IPV within this patient population.[23] Clinicians should suspend assumptions about "perpetrator" and "victim" roles based on gender stereotypes.

Sexually transmitted infection prevention

Counseling on prevention of STIs should be undertaken in all adolescent and young women less than 25 years of age, and all high-risk adults (intermittent/absent condom usage, multiple sex partners, those who have sex with members of high-risk groups: sex and gender minorities; commercial sex workers; intravenous drug users), to prevent STI acquisition.[22] Patients should be asked about their sexual behaviors, including penetrative, oral, and anal sex.[24] Patients should also be asked about their sexual partners, including number and sex/gender, and assumptions should be suspended before questioning. Providers should discuss condom usage, including barriers to condom usage, and patient agency in requesting condom usage from their partners. Providers should be aware of the ways in which IPV and trauma may impact a patient's agency in negotiating for safer sex, and appropriate referrals should be provided if appropriate. If appropriate, preexposure prophylaxis should be discussed depending on the risk factors for HIV acquisition.[22]

Contraception

Contraception should be discussed at every preventative care visit starting at age 13 years, regardless of whether sexual activity has started. Patients should be counseled on all available methods, starting with the most effective forms first.[24] Long-acting reversible contraceptives (LARCs) (eg, Nexplanon, intrauterine device [IUD], Depo-Provera) are appropriate choices in this age group, owing to the safety of LARCs and increased efficacy of LARCs compared with short-term contraceptives.[25] Other options, including all combined hormonal methods, should also be discussed. Barrier contraception should always be encouraged as a secondary method of contraception to increase contraceptive efficacy and prevent STI transmission.[25] Adolescents and young adults may have misconceptions regarding various methods of contraception, and time should be taken to address misconceptions and concerns that patients have.[25] Patients should be protected from reproductive coercion, and all steps should be taken to encourage patient autonomy over reproductive health.[25]

Contraception counseling should not be limited to adolescents and young adults and should be discussed with all persons with the possibility of conception, regardless of current sexual activity.[25] Discussion of side effects should be undertaken, as well as any barriers to care or misconceptions regarding contraception in the adult population. Emergency contraception should be discussed ahead of time with all patients, including adolescents.[25]

Care should also be taken to consider the need for contraceptive counseling in gender minority patients in whom sexual activity includes sperm and oocyte. Hormone therapy is not a form of contraceptive, and so fertility goals should be discussed.[26] All patients should be counseled on using barrier methods to prevent STIs in addition to pregnancy; however, if additional contraception is desired, patients should be counseled that testosterone therapy is not a contraindication to using estrogen-containing contraceptives.[26] In addition, patients should be informed on alternate progestin-only methods like the progestin IUD, progestin implant, or progestin injection.[26]

Recommended cancer screenings

All patients should be advised regarding recommended screenings, including Papanicolaou test, mammogram, etc. In the case of HIV+ gay and bisexual men, anal Papanicolaou test should also be discussed and shared decision making used to determine the risk versus benefit of testing.[23] Transgender patients who have anatomic structures consistent with their gender assigned at birth should be counseled on appropriate cancer screenings as well (eg, transgender man with uterine cervix should be offered Papanicolaou test).[23] Care should be taken to assess any barriers to screening or misconceptions regarding screening that the patient may possess. If misconceptions are identified, patient education should be provided to correct these beliefs.

Adolescent care and confidentiality

Adolescents should be counseled on their rights to confidential medical care regarding sexual health and contraception, because fears regarding confidentiality are a major barrier to gynecologic care in this patient population.[25] Practitioners should be aware of individual state laws regarding confidentiality in this population.[25] Adolescents and parents should be informed of the reasons for a break in confidentiality (concerns for safety of patient, safety of others, child abuse, etc.). Providers should encourage open communication between the parent and child; however, this should not be a requirement for providing care to the minor patient.[25]

Sexual function

Providers should ask about sexual dysfunction at every annual preventative care visit.[27] Women may experience concerns about sexual dysfunction, including dyspareunia, sexual interest, or ability to reach orgasm, and may be uncomfortable addressing these concerns with their provider.[27] Care should be taken to suspend assumptions about sexual activity and the sex and gender of partners, and providers should ask questions about sexuality in an open-ended manner. If a sexual concern is identified, providers should provide counseling about the multifactorial nature of sexual dysfunction, including relationship factors, mental health, fatigue and stress, and physiologic changes, and that the pathway to relieving sexual dysfunction may take time.[27] From there, follow-up can be scheduled to take a detailed history determining the underlying cause, and treatment options including referral for sex therapy, individual or couples counseling, pelvic floor physical therapy, or medication.[27] For patients experiencing sexual pain secondary to atrophic vaginitis, the provider should counsel on the use of lubricants and vaginal moisturizers to improve comfort with penetrative intercourse, in addition to prescription treatment options.[28] Similarly, the importance of using lubrication should be discussed with transgender women who have undergone surgical creation of a neovagina, due to the tendency for sexual pain if lubricant is neglected.[28]

SUMMARY

As health care providers, it is of the utmost importance to obtain detailed sexual histories on our patients. Ensuring we have taken an unbiased and comprehensive approach to this important aspect of our patient encounter will allow us to provide better care for our patient's overall health. Screening for STIs, discussing recommended USPSTF cancer screenings, and providing recommendations as per the CDC in regard to vaccinations for viruses with potential for sexual transmission should be routine parts of the encounter based on the patient's age and overall health status. In addition, taking time to counsel patients of all ages on topics including IPV, contraception, sexual dysfunction, and STI transmission should be approached in ways that patients are comfortable discussing and may reveal insights into the patient's overall mental and physical health status.

CLINICS CARE POINTS

- The 5 Ps for obtaining a sexual history include "partners, practices, prevention against pregnancy, protection against sexually transmitted infections, past history of sexually transmitted infections."[29]

- USPSTF recommends starting Papanicolaou tests at age 21 years regardless of sexual activity[8]; "the majority of patients with an abnormal Pap before age 21 will have regression of most lesions."[8,21]

- HPV is the most common viral STI in the United States.[1,21] Owing to the increasing number of HPV vaccinations being given to patients, recent data suggests that there is developing herd immunity to HPV.[21]

- Many transgender people have not had genital affirmation surgery and retain their natal sex organs; therefore it is important to make appropriate cancer screening recommendations based off of their natal sex.[30]
- Sexual dysfunction is a common problem but often not readily disclosed by the patient. In aging men, "the most common type of sexual dysfunction is erectile dysfunction, and the most common etiology is vascular disease. In aging women, sexual dysfunction is often multifactorial, including lack of estrogen causing vaginal dryness and lack of testosterone decreasing libido."[31]

DISCLOSURE

The authors have nothing to disclose.

REFERENCES

1. Centers for Disease Control and Prevention. Sexually transmitted disease surveillance 2018. Available at: https://www.cdc.gov/std/stats18/default.htm. Accessed March 3, 2021.
2. American Academy of Family Physicians. Sexually transmitted infections (STI) survey report 2019. Accessed March 3, 2021.
3. American Academy of Family Physicians. Adolescent health clinical recommendations & guidelines. Available at: www.aafp.org/patient-care/browse/topics. tag-adolescent-health.html. Accessed March 22, 2021.
4. Human Rights Campaign. Transgender people and HIV: what we know. Available at: www.hrc.org/resources/transgender-people-and-hiv-what-we-know. Accessed March 3, 2021.
5. Centers for Disease Control and Prevention. Sexually transmitted diseases treatment guidelines. Screening 2015. Available at: www.cdc.gov/std/tg2015/qa/ screening-qa.htm. Accessed March 3, 2021.
6. Partnership for Prevention. Take charge of your sexual health: what you need to know about preventive services. Washington, DC: Partnership for Prevention; 2014.
7. Saraiya M, Unger ER, Thompson TD, et al. U.S. assessment of HPV types in cancers: implications for current and 9-valent HPV vaccines. J Natl Cancer Inst 2015; 107(6):djv086.
8. Rerucha CM, Caro R, Wheeler V. Cervical cancer screening. Am Fam Physician 2018. Available at: https://www.aafp.org/afp/2018/0401/p441.html. Accessed March 15, 2021.
9. McGinley KF, Hey W, Sussman DO, et al. Human papillomavirus testing in men. J Am Osteopath Assoc 2011. Available at: https://jaoa.org/article.aspx? articleid=2094178. Accessed March 15, 2021.
10. Hepatitis B. World Health Organization 2020. Available at: https://www.who.int/ news-room/fact-sheets/detail/hepatitis-b. Accessed March 12, 2021.
11. Sarah S, Wester C, et al. CDC recommendations for Hepatitis C screening among adults 2020. Available at: https://www.cdc.gov/mmwr/volumes/69/rr/pdfs/ rr6902a1-H.pdf. Accessed March 15, 2021.
12. CDC call to action: let's work together to stem the tide of rising syphilis in the U.S. centers for disease control and prevention. Available at: https://npin.cdc.gov/ publication/cdc-call-action-lets-work. Accessed March 2, 2021.
13. American Academy of Family Physicians. Clinical preventive service recommendation. HIV screening, adolescents, and adults. Available at: www.aafp.org/

patient-care/clinical-recommendations/all/hiv-screening.html. Accessed March 14, 2021.

14. American Academy of Family Physicians. Screening for sexually transmitted infections practice manual from scientific activities. 2019. Accessed March 2021.

15. Ask the experts about human papillomavirus (HPV) vaccines - CDC experts answer Q&As. Immunize.org. 2020. Available at: https://www.immunize.org/askexperts/experts_hpv.asp. Accessed March 23, 2021.

16. Ask the experts: hepatitis A vaccines. Immunize.org. 2020. Available at: https://www.immunize.org/askexperts/experts_hepa.asp. Accessed March 23, 2021.

17. Ask the experts: hepatitis B vaccines. Immunize.org. 2020. Available at: https://www.immunize.org/askexperts/experts_hepb.asp. Accessed March 23, 2021.

18. Vaccine information statement | Hepatitis A | VIS | CDC. Hepatitis A VIS. 2020. Available at: https://www.cdc.gov/vaccines/hcp/vis/vis-statements/hep-a.html. Accessed March 23, 2021.

19. Vaccine information statement|hepatitis B|VIS|CDC. Hepatitis B VIS. Available at: https://www.cdc.gov/vaccines/hcp/vis/vis-statements/hep-b.html. Accessed March 23, 2021.

20. Vaccine Information Statement|HPV|VIS|CDC. HPV (Human Papillomavirus) VIS. 2019. Available at: https://www.cdc.gov/vaccines/hcp/vis/vis-statements/hpv.html. Accessed March 23, 2021.

21. Graber M, Ray B, Wilbur J. Graber and Wilbur's family medicine examination and board review. 5th edition. United States: MCGRAW-HILL EDUCATION; 2020. Section 15.

22. ACOG Foundation. Recommendations for well-woman care clinical summary tables. Women's preventative services initiative 2021. Available at: www.womenspreventivehealth.org/wp-content/uploads/WPSI_ClinicalSummaryTables_2021Updates.pdf. Accessed March 14, 2021.

23. Smalley KB, et al. LGBT health: meeting the needs of gender and sexual minorities. Springer Publishing Company, LLC; 2018.

24. Altarum Institute. Sexual health and your patients: provider's guide. National Coalition for Sexual Health 2016. Available at: nationalcoalitionforsexualhealth.org/tools/for-healthcare-providers/document/Provider-Guide_2021.pdf. Accessed March 9, 2021.

25. Committee on Adolescent Health Care, Gerancher KK. Counseling adolescents about contraception. American College of Obstetrics and Gynecologists 2017. Available at: www.acog.org/en/Clinical/Clinical%20Guidance/Committee%20Opinion/Articles/2017/08/Counseling%20Adolescents%20About%20Contraception. Accessed March 3, 2021.

26. Committee on Gynecologic Practice and Committee on Health Care for Underserved Women, et al. Health care for transgender and gender diverse individuals 2021. Available at: www.acog.org/en/Clinical/Clinical%20Guidance/Committee%20Opinion/Articles/2021/03/Health%20Care%20for%20Transgender%20and%20Gender%20Diverse%20Individuals. Accessed March 4, 2021.

27. Shifren JL. Overview of sexual dysfunction in women: epidemiology, risk factors, and evaluation. UpToDate 2020. Available at: www.uptodate.com/contents/overview-of-sexual-dysfunction-in-women-epidemiology-risk-factors-and-evaluation?search=sexual+dysfunction&source=search_result&selectedTitle=2~150&usage_type=default&display_rank=2. Accessed March 9, 2021.

28. Shifren JL. Overview of sexual dysfunction: management. UpToDate 2020. Available at: www.uptodate.com/contents/overview-of-sexual-dysfunction-in-women-management?search=sexual+dysfunction&source=search_result&selected

Title=3~150&usage_type=default&display_rank=3#H3703806368. Accessed March 9, 2021.

29. StatPearls. Sexually transmitted infections. Sexually transmitted infection. 2020. Available at: https://www.statpearls.com/ArticleLibrary/viewarticle/28956. Accessed March 25, 2021.

30. Yehia BR, Makadon HJ. Lesbian, gay, bisexual, and transgender (LGBT) health. In: Jameson J, Fauci AS, Kasper DL, et al. eds. Harrison's principles of internal medicine, 20e. McGraw-Hill. Available at: https://accessmedicine.mhmedical. com/content.aspx?bookid=2129&sectionid=192288190. Accessed March 25, 2021.

31. Waring E, Gentili A, Godschalk M. Sexual health & dysfunction. In: Walter LC, Chang A, Chen P, et al. eds. Current diagnosis & treatment geriatrics, 3e. McGraw-Hill; Accessed March 25, 2021.

Vaccines

Andrew P. Chastain, MSPAS, PA-C[a],*, Matéa M. Rippe, MPAS, PA-C[b],
Tia M. Solh, MT(ASCP), MSPAS, PA-C[c], Jennifer Simms Zorn, DMS, PA-C[d]

KEYWORDS

- Barriers • Current guidelines • Provider education • Strategies • Vaccination
- Vaccine • Vaccine uptake • Immunity

KEY POINTS

- When discussing, ordering, or administering vaccinations to patients, it is incumbent upon health care providers to consider and understand the different types of vaccines and how each works.
- Providers must have literacy, as it pertains to current clinical guidelines when discussing, ordering, or administering vaccinations to patients.
- Prescribers must take into account the barriers that exist in preventing optimal vaccine uptake and develop strategies to help patients in overcoming these barriers.

INTRODUCTION

The development of vaccines against infectious diseases is one of the most significant scientific advances in human history. Vaccines have completely eradicated infections such as polio and smallpox, and nearly eliminated others such as measles, mumps, rubella, diphtheria, tetanus, and pertussis.[1,2] As a result, millions of lives have been preserved. And while rates of immunization in the United States have continued to rise, exceeding 90% for children entering kindergarten, opportunities exist to improve upon these rates if we are to meet the objectives as outlined in the Healthy People 2030 goals.[3,4] The key to this is for health care providers to develop and maintain vaccination literacy through continued medical education. Understanding the types of vaccines available and how each works to activate the patient's immune system is key. In addition, care must be placed on continuing to stay abreast of the most recent clinical guidelines. Lastly, providers must take into account the barriers that exist in preventing optimal vaccine uptake and develop strategies to help patients in overcoming these barriers.

[a] Butler University, 4600 Sunset Avenue, Indianapolis, IN 46208, USA; [b] 401 E 34th Street, Indianapolis, IN 46205, USA; [c] Department of Physician Assistant Studies, South College - Atlanta Campus, 2600 Century Parkway Northeast, Atlanta, GA 30345, USA; [d] Butler University, 4600 Sunset Avenue, Indianapolis, IN 46208, USA
* Corresponding author.
E-mail address: achastain@butler.edu

Physician Assist Clin 7 (2022) 127–139
https://doi.org/10.1016/j.cpha.2021.08.004
2405-7991/22/© 2021 Elsevier Inc. All rights reserved.
physicianassistant.theclinics.com

VACCINE PATHOPHYSIOLOGY AND PHARMACOLOGY

When considering the pathophysiology of vaccines, understanding the types of vaccines is critical to a basic understanding of the pathophysiology and pharmacology related to their utilization. Vaccines are categorized into groups often based on the immunogenic components that are introduced: live attenuated vaccines, inactivated vaccines, subunit vaccines which may include protein, toxoid vaccines, and polysaccharide and polysaccharide conjugate vaccines.[5–10] The vaccine may include an adjuvant to increase the immune response of vaccines that are not live-attenuated. Aluminum-containing adjuvants (Alum) have been used since the 1930s and is the most common adjuvant used.[11] Currently, aluminum salts are the only FDA-approved adjuvants. One way the Alum increases the immune response is by the ability to activate the innate immune response. This independent activation of an immune response is likely a contributing factor.[5,6]

The various types of vaccines introduce at least a part of a disease-causing agent and are discussed in the following list:

- Live attenuated vaccines
  - This vaccine type introduces a live virus or bacteria that has been weakened to cause a very limited infection. This vaccination type is more likely to produce lifelong immunity which differs from the nonliving vaccines which have a shorter duration and frequently require boosters for continued immunity.[5,6] However, individuals who are immunocompromised and receive a live attenuated vaccine may be at risk for increased replication of the pathogen, and administration of live-attenuated vaccines should be considered carefully in this population.[5]
- Inactivated vaccine
  - These are entire pathogens that have been inactivated by a process that may include exposure to chemicals, heat, or radiation, and therefore cannot cause disease or reactivate.
- Subunit vaccines
  - This type has fewer antigens and contributes to a lower reaction. The subunit vaccines contain fragments created depending on the type of subunit.
- Protein antigens
  - This vaccine may be purified or created by recombinant DNA techniques to produce the protein.
- Toxoid vaccines
  - This type of vaccine destroys the activity of the toxin produced by the bacteria and uses that to cause the immunologic response in the patient.
- Viral-Like Particles (VLPs)
  - These are viral proteins that assemble similar to the virus but are not infectious because only the proteins are present and not the viral genome.
- Polysaccharide vaccines
  - These vaccines are not significantly immunogenic, though the initial intent was to assist in recognition of the protective polysaccharide covering certain infectious agents. The newer vaccines use a carrier protein to change the immune response to a dependent T-cell process. The production requires an attachment of a protein to the purified polysaccharides.[5–9]

Vaccines are designed for the body to create an immune response to provide long-term immunity in a person by inducing both the innate and the antigen-specific immune responses.[5] The desire is not only to protect individuals with vaccines but also to develop herd immunity in this process so there are enough people immunized in a population to protect those who have not had the immunization as the risk of an outbreak is low. This is a critical component to consider as there are always individuals in the population that are contraindicated for some vaccines at different times including age, pregnancy, or anaphylactic reactions to components. The power of this herd immunity was demonstrated in the country of Gambia where Haemophilus Influenza B (Hib) was eliminated with a vaccination rate of 70% of the population.[5,9] It is of note that the threshold for herd immunity varies depending on the contagiousness of the disease, the efficacy of its vaccine, and the number in the community with immunity either with vaccination or developed from surviving an infection.

Once the form of a disease-causing agent has been introduced via the administration of the vaccine, antigen-presenting cells engulf and process antigens to present with the major histocompatibility complexes. Most often the utilization of T helper or CD4+ T cells is involved in the process after the presentation of the antigen, but there are some instances when the antigen will stimulate the B-lymphocyte directly.[11] The T helper cell will then stimulate the B-lymphocyte to produce antibodies. Some B-lymphocytes will become plasma forming cells which then assist in the activation of the humoral and cellular immune response. This includes antibody production, macrophage stimulation, CD8+ T cell activation, and memory cell development. Antibody production begins as IgM and then will produce IgG antibodies. The antibodies themselves may function as antitoxins, lysins, prevention of adhesion of bacteria as well as preventing the reproduction of viruses. With the ability for the body to complete the immune response with the vaccine, there is an increased and more rapid response to future encounters.[10,11] Vaccines may require a second dose or a booster during one's lifetime to maintain or improve immunity by reactivating their immune system. This may be more commonly needed in the vaccines that are not live attenuated vaccines.

VACCINATION RECOMMENDATIONS
Current Guidelines

Immunizations are paramount in preventing infections in individuals of all ages and are universally recommended as a top-tier preventative health measure.[12,13] All health care providers must be familiar with the indicated vaccines for each age and risk group to ensure adequate coverage against vaccine-preventable infections. In the United States, the Advisory Committee on Immunization Practices (ACIP) is charged with developing and disseminating vaccine recommendations and policies, and does so based on the best quality of evidence available regarding disease epidemiology, the burden of disease, and vaccine efficacy and safety.[14] All recommendations become official following approval by the director of the Centers for Disease Control and Prevention (CDC), which are then published in the Morbidity and Mortality Weekly Report, as well as in journals of collaborating medical societies.[14] The ACIP issues 2 immunization schedule recommendations annually: one for children and adolescents through 18 years of age and one for adults aged 19 and older. A modified summary of the recommended routine vaccinations for immunocompetent individuals by an infectious agent, age, and other considerations is shown in **Table 1**.[15,16] For a complete summary, including detailed recommendations for specific chronic medical conditions as well as catch-up schedules, please refer to the current CDC vaccination schedules located on its Web site.

Special Populations

Vaccination recommendations for specific populations that differ from the recommended routine vaccination schedules are discussed in the following sections:

Table 1
Summary of recommended routine vaccinations across the lifespan

Recommended Vaccine	Associated Infectious Agents	Recommended Age Groups	Considerations
Hep B	Hepatitis B virus	3-dose series starting at birth, 1–2 mo of age, and 6–18 mo	For infants born to mothers who are positive for Hep B surface antigen, administer Hep B immune globulin in addition to series.
Diphtheria, tetanus, and acellular pertussis (DTaP)	Corynebacterium diphtheriae; Clostridium tetani; Bordetella pertussis	4-dose series starting at 2 mo of age; 4 mo; 6 mo; 15–18 mo. Booster dose given at 4–6 y.	Future doses are contraindicated if encephalopathy develops within 7 d of a DTaP dose.
Hib	Haemophilus influenzae type B	3-dose series starting at 2 mo of age; 4 mo; 12–15 mo	4-dose series may be given instead at 2, 4, 6, and 12–15 mo.
Pneumococcal conjugate vaccine (PCV13)	Streptococcus pneumoniae; 13 serotypes	4-dose series starting at 2 mo of age; 4 mo; 6 mo; and 12–15 mo 1 dose at age 65 y or older.	Patients at increased risk may receive earlier and additional doses.
Inactivated poliovirus (IPV)	Poliovirus	4-dose series starting at 2 mo of age; 4 mo; 6–18 mo; and 4–6 y.	Routine vaccination of adults is not indicated unless traveling to countries with endemic polio.
Rotavirus (RV): RV1 (2 dose series); or RV5 (3-dose series)	Rotavirus	2 mo and 4 mo of age for 2-dose series; 2, 4, and 6 mo of age for 3-dose series	History of rotavirus gastroenteritis is not a contraindication.
Inactivated influenza vaccine (IIV)	Influenza virus	Annually beginning at age 6 mo	Children age 6 mo to 8 y who have received fewer than 2 influenza vaccine doses will require 2 doses. Patients with severe egg allergies should receive vaccine in a supervised health care setting.
Measles, mumps, rubella (MMR)	Measles (rubeola) virus; mumps virus; rubella virus	2-dose series at 12–15 mo and 4–6 y old.	1 or 2 doses should be given beginning at age 19 y if no evidence of immunity.

Vaccine	Organism	Schedule	Notes
Varicella (VAR)	*Varicella-zoster virus*	2-dose series at 12–15 mo and 4–6 y old.	Varicella vaccine may be given in combination with MMR in children >47 mo of age. 2-dose series should be given at age 19 y if no evidence of immunity.
Hepatitis A (HepA)	*Hepatitis A virus*	2-dose series beginning at 12 mo of age; preferably before 24 mo.	Adults with risk factors may receive 2-dose series of HepA or 3-dose series of combined HepA and HepB.
Tetanus, diphtheria, and acellular pertussis (Tdap)	*Clostridium tetani; Corynebacterium diphtheriae; Bordetella pertussis*	Age 11–12 y; age 19 y and older; then Td (tetanus, diphtheria) or Tdap every 10 y	Td may be indicated in wound management if >5 y since last dose.
Human papillomavirus (HPV)	*Human papillomavirus types 6, 11, 16, 18, 31, 33, 45, 52, and 58.*	2-dose series beginning at age 11–12 y 3-dose series recommended if starting dose given at age 15 y.	Start at age 9 y if history of sexual abuse or assault. May begin 2 or 3 dose series at age 19 y if no prior. Not generally indicated after age 26 y.
Meningococcal (MenACWY-D and MenACWY-CRM)	*Neisseria meningitidis serogroups A,C,W,Y*	2-dose series at 11–12 y and at 16 y	May be administered earlier in high-risk children. Adults at continued high-risk for meningococcal disease should receive additional doses.
Meningococcal B (MenB)	*Neisseria meningitidis serogroup B*	2 dose series starting at age 16–18 y (preferred)	Booster doses recommended for immunocompromised after completion of series.
Pneumococcal polysaccharide (PPSV23)	*Streptococcus pneumoniae; 23 serotypes*	4-dose series starting at 2 mo, 4 mo, 6 mo, and 12–15 mo 1 dose ages 19–64 y with chronic medical conditions; 1 dose at age 65 y or older.	≥ 65: PPSV23 should be given 1 y after PCV 13 and ≥ 5 y after the previous PPSV23.
Recombinant zoster vaccine (RZV)	*Varicella-zoster virus*	2-dose series beginning at age 50 y	Administer regardless of previous herpes zoster or history of ZVL.
Live zoster vaccine (ZVL)	*Varicella-zoster virus*	1 dose may be given at age 60 y or older instead of RZV series (if no prior vaccination).	RZV preferred over ZVL.

Pregnant women

Owing to the possible risk of fetal injury, live attenuated vaccines are not recommended in pregnancy. Inactivated vaccines should be administered as indicated, and if benefits outweigh potential risks. To foster passive antibody transfer to the fetus, all pregnant women should receive the annual inactivated influenza vaccine seasonally, and a Tdap dose preferably between 27 and 36 weeks of gestation. The HPV vaccine is currently not recommended in pregnancy.[17]

Preterm infants

Most infants born before 37 weeks' gestation may receive the same routinely recommended vaccinations at the same chronologic age, dose, and schedule as for full-term infants. For preterm infants born weighing less than 2000 g, the first dose of the hepatitis B vaccine administered at birth will not count toward the series, which will start at age 1 month instead.[18]

Breastfeeding women

All vaccine types, including inactivated, recombinant, subunit, polysaccharide, and conjugate vaccines, as well as toxoids, have been found to pose no risk to breastfeeding women or their infants.[17] Breastfeeding women may also receive all live vaccines as appropriate, except for the smallpox vaccine, because of the theoretic risk of contact transmission to the infant. Vaccination for yellow fever should also be avoided unless the mother is traveling to an endemic area.

The immunocompromised

In general, individuals who are severely immunocompromised with conditions such as AIDS (acquired immunodeficiency syndrome), congenital immunodeficiencies, hematologic malignancies, solid tumor malignancies, anatomic or functional asplenia, solid organ transplant, or are taking immunosuppressants should not receive live vaccinations because of the risk of viral replication and subsequent blunted or lack of host response. Detailed recommendations regarding the administration of inactivated vaccines vary per condition and severity of immunosuppression and are beyond the scope of this article.[19]

BARRIERS TO VACCINE UPTAKE

When we consider what prevents our patients from reaching full vaccination status, the barriers are numerous and wide-ranging. A recent meta-analysis of 43 studies on the subject, conducted by Thomson, and colleagues, distilled down and categorized the most frequently identified barriers to vaccine uptake and produced a practical taxonomy that classifies these determinants into 5 categories. Known as "The 5A's," these determinants are awareness, activation, acceptance, access, and affordability.[20] We will use these categories as a construct to further explore the barriers that may prevent our patients from becoming fully vaccinated.

Awareness

Awareness, when considered as a barrier to vaccine uptake, is the patient's knowledge of the need for and timing of recommended vaccines. In addition, this can also include the patient's understanding of the benefits and risks associated with the vaccine.[20] This lack of awareness and knowledge about vaccinations is often associated with suboptimal vaccination rates, particularly in marginalized populations.[21] As recently as 2008, a North Carolina study showed that only about 19% of

African Americans surveyed had ever heard of the HPV vaccine.[22,23] Lack of health literacy can act as a barrier to achieving optimal vaccination status in the community.

Activation

Activation, when considered as a barrier to vaccine uptake, is defined as those actions that encourage patients/parents to accept vaccination. It centers on the notion that patients are more often vaccinated if they are either reminded or prompted by their provider, or if they are required to do so to maintain employment.[20] Failure to set up systems to optimize practice or provider activation in our communities leads to diminished childhood immunization.[3]

Acceptance

Acceptance, when considered as a barrier to vaccine uptake, is defined as the likelihood a patient/parent will accept or refuse a vaccine. Reasons for variance in acceptance are based on a multitude of factors such as concern for vaccine safety/efficacy, religious beliefs, political views, mistrust of the medical/pharmaceutical industry, and even that specific vaccines might encourage sexual activity.[20] Barriers that are classified in this category are the most commonly researched.[20]

Safety Concerns

Safety concerns among patients/parents continue to prevent optimal vaccination status in the community. In fact, despite best efforts to the contrary, there remain those who question the safety and necessity of vaccinations.[24] Twenty years on from the publication of the Wakefield paper,[25] and its subsequent retraction, parental concerns persist that there is a causal relationship between vaccinations and autism despite a multitude of evidence that proves that this is not the case. There has been no epidemiologic or accepted scientific study that shows that either thimerosal or the MMR vaccine causes autism.[26]

There remain some who worry that the current vaccination schedule, containing protection against 14 vaccine-preventable diseases over the first 24 months of life, will overwhelm the newborn/infant immune system. The overall bacterial and viral material contained in today's modern vaccines is far less as compared with those given as recently as the 1980s.[26] Of course, most vaccines contain far fewer than 100 antigens (eg, the hepatitis B, diphtheria, and tetanus vaccines each contains 1 antigen), so the estimated number of vaccines to which a child could respond is conservative. But using this estimate, we would predict that if 11 vaccines were given to infants at one time, then about 0.1% of the immune system would be 'used up.'[27]

Religious/Personal Beliefs

Another subset of patients/parents cites religious or personal beliefs as a reason why they will not consent to the recommended vaccination schedule. Many (but not all) object based upon religious beliefs and are opposed to vaccines that are derived from or cultivated through the use of aborted fetal tissue.[28] Included among these are vaccination preparations for rubella, varicella, hepatitis A, adenovirus, and one preparation of the rabies vaccine. In addition, others cite a personal right to refuse vaccinations for themselves or their children. In one study of parents who refused mandatory school vaccination requirements for their children, 47% agreed that they should have the right to do so.[29] In response to this, 47 states allow for a religious exemption to the accepted vaccination requirements, and 17 offer exemption based on personal beliefs.[30,31] These nonmedical exemptions tend to be regional and associated with increased outbreaks of vaccine-preventable diseases.[32]

Specific Barriers to Human Papillomavirus Uptake

There appear to be unique barriers to the uptake of the vaccination for human papillomavirus (HPV). These barriers appear to be multifactorial, but up to 20% of parents report being concerned that the vaccine may affect young women's sexual behavior.[33] Multiple US and Canadian studies have shown that there is not a correlation between receiving the HPV vaccine and engagement in risky sexual behavior.[34,35]

Mistrust of the Medical/Pharmaceutical Professions

Another barrier in discussing vaccination acceptance, among those who are inclined to refuse, are those who harbor a distrust of the medical and/or pharmaceutical industries. Those who cite this distrust typically fall into 1 of 2 categories. The first are those who see widespread vaccination as a means of generating revenue for the clinician, medical practice, health system, and/or the pharmaceutical industry. The second are those members of marginalized groups whose distrust is based on a long history of health care inequity, discrimination, and even medical experimentation.[36,37]

Access to and Affordability of Vaccines

The last barrier to vaccination uptake surrounds access and affordability of vaccines. Although the CDC's Vaccines For Children (VFC) program eliminates the direct cost of vaccines to those who are eligible, the opportunity cost of time away (eg, from work, from another children's care) remains a barrier. As it pertains to access, one study researching uptake of the influenza vaccine found significantly lower uptake for non-Hispanic Black, Hispanic, and American Indian/Native Alaskan adults when compared with their non-Hispanic White adult counterparts.[38,39] In addition, those patients who are foreign-born—particularly in countries where vaccine-preventable diseases are endemic—are both at increased risk of premigration and subsequent exposures, while also having limited access and interaction with health care providers.[40]

STRATEGIES TO IMPROVE VACCINE UPTAKE
Provider Education

To overcome barriers to vaccination uptake, providers must first commit to the process of self-education regarding vaccination in their clinical setting. This includes a sound understanding of vaccine efficacy and terminology, individual obstacles to full vaccination, and the availability of accurate information and resources within the community.[41] When put into practice, this information must also be able to translate into a clear and meaningful message for patients. These conversations require intentional time and adequate preparation. Such preparation may involve individual research, reflection, and potentially formal training. One study, in particular, demonstrated significant improvement in the ability of students to confidently lead a conversation with a vaccine-hesitant patient after a brief training by the American Pharmacist Association's certification program.[42] Engagement in such formal training may assist providers as they frequently apply information in a strategic context with patients.

Continuous Dialogue

Fruitful dialogue concerning vaccination significance cannot be accomplished within the time frame of one patient visit. To address barriers to vaccination, providers must promote transmission of ideas and establish rapport at every appointment. By maintaining an open conversation, clinicians may continue developing the patient-provider relationship while gaining an understanding of patient concerns. The clinician is then better prepared to provide individualized instruction that targets misconceptions or sources of misinformation.[43] Using a model of continuous conversation, a provider may also create opportunities for educating patients on vaccine terminology, efficacy, and importance. This requires using time intentionally during the patient visit and leaving space for questions and continued conversation. To keep the message clear and concise, the World Health Organization recommends clinicians use basic facts, make clear warnings, explain erroneous myths, and present graphics as key components of the discussion.[43] One method to avoid in continued conversation is providing written, corrective information. Unless specifically requested by patients, the provision of such written materials has been shown to reduce intent to vaccinate. When using this strategy, providers assume their patients will trust the given information, while a patient's major concern with vaccination may already be grounded in mistrust.[41]

Another benefit of continuous dialogue regarding vaccinations is that more opportunities are created for patient reminder and recall interventions. Reminder interventions are focused on educating patients or caregivers which vaccines are coming next, whereas recall interventions provide notification of which vaccines are overdue.[3,44] These interventions have been proven to increase vaccine uptake by helping to simplify seemingly complex vaccination schedules. Maintaining a more narrowed focus on the vaccination schedule avoids overwhelming the patient while keeping them informed of the more immediate steps in their plan of care.

Empathic Approach

Medical providers may reason that the best way to combat vaccine hesitancy is through statistics and logic, but there is an increasing amount of data showing the efficacy of emotional appeal in vaccination discussions. One of the most readily available examples of this theory is well-meaning parents who have been dissuaded from vaccinating their children after hearing compelling theories about the harms of vaccination. Using the same emotional petition, many parents repeal their decision when confronted with the potentially life-altering consequences of vaccination refusal.[41] To initiate an emotive discussion with a vaccine-hesitant individual, it is best to acknowledge a common goal of optimizing the patient's health. In addition, it is beneficial to verbally affirm their efforts to make informed decisions and advocate for their health.[43] In situations where patients come with opinions shaped by the plethora of conflicting information found on the Internet, it is especially important to support their investment and be willing to patiently discuss their findings using the model of continuous dialogue. Such a continuous discussion may also be supplemented with anecdotal evidence of vaccine safety and efficacy. Providers who share their own experiences, reasoning, and choices regarding vaccinating themselves and their families are more likely to persuade vaccine-hesitant individuals by the emotional appeal of personal endorsement.[45]

Community Outreach

Some of the most effective and lasting improvements to vaccine uptake occur at the community level. Studies have shown that community-wide involvement in this process is the surest way to reach a large number of individuals. However, provoking change at the community level also requires the largest amount of time, effort, and resources. Several strategies of community outreach have been studied and many have proven effective in their efforts to improve vaccine uptake. One method involves implementing walk-in and extended hours at clinics while offering vaccines free of charge. Such clinics have shown to be very effective, although straining on resources and clinicians.[3] Another method involves computerized immunization registries, where clinical practices and the state can maintain records of children who have not been receiving consistent medical care and/or lack proper preventative care. Using this impactful platform, unvaccinated or undervaccinated children are identified, and reminders are created for both parents and providers to pursue vaccinations for those individuals.[3] This helps to target at-risk children and improve vaccination uptake within the community as a whole. A third effective method of improving community vaccine uptake is collaboration between health care organizations, daycares, pharmacies, and other social organizations to promote vaccine distribution in pre-existing community programs.[3] This method is much less labor-intensive and financially burdensome because it operates as an addition to pre-established programs rather than an independent service.

SUMMARY

Proper preventative medicine is an essential component of quality health care. As more patients and caregivers personally seek out credible information to make informed decisions, it is imperative for providers to be aware of current guidelines, barriers to proper care, and strategies to overcome those barriers. Increasing vaccination uptake is a single but impactful step toward the achievement of comprehensive preventative medicine.

CLINICS CARE POINTS

- Vaccination to preventable disease is a key to preventive medicine, and to maintain or build upon current vaccination rates, providers must continue to stay informed about:
  ○ The types of vaccines available and their constituent components.
  ○ The mechanism by which each vaccine works.
  ○ Current clinical guidelines based on age and patient risk.

- Barriers to vaccine uptake can be challenging to overcome. Being aware of what prevents a patient from being optimally vaccinated requires patience, openness, and rapport.

- Creating a continuous, educated, and empathic discourse with patients and parents about the importance of vaccinations is the best strategy for overcoming barriers to vaccine hesitancy/refusal.

DISCLOSURE

The authors have nothing to disclose.

REFERENCES

1. Rappuoli R, Mandl CW, Black S, et al. Vaccines for the twenty-first century society. Nat Rev Immunol 2011;11(12):865–72. Erratum in: Nat Rev Immunol. 2012 Mar;12(3):225.
2. Mishra RPN, Oviedo-Orta E, Prachi P, et al. Vaccines and antibiotic resistance. Curr Opin Microbiol 2012;15(5):596–602.
3. Frew PM, Lutz CS. Interventions to increase pediatric vaccine uptake: an overview of recent findings. Hum Vaccin Immunother 2017;13(11):2503–11.
4. Office of Disease Prevention and Health Promotion. Vaccination. Healthy People 2030. U.S. Department of Health and Human Services. Available at: https://

health.gov/healthypeople/objectives-and-data/browse-objectives/vaccination. Accessed November 11, 2020.

5. Vetter V, Denizer G, Friedland LR, et al. Understanding modern-day vaccines: what you need to know. Ann Med 2018;50(2):110–20.

6. Pulendran B, Ahmed R. Immunological mechanisms of vaccination. Nat Immunol 2011;12(6):509–17.

7. Plotkin SA. Vaccines, vaccination, and vaccinology. J Infect Dis 2003;187(9): 1349–59.

8. Understanding how vaccines work. Centers for Disease Control and Prevention website. 2020. Available at: https://www.cdc.gov/vaccines/hcp/conversations/understanding-vacc-work.html. Accessed January 6, 2020.

9. How vaccines work. PublicHealth.org. Available at: https://www.publichealth.org/public-awareness/understanding-vaccines/vaccines-work/. Accessed January 9, 2020.

10. Justiz Vaillant AA, Grella MJ. Vaccine (vaccination). In: StatPearls [internet]. Treasure Island (FL): StatPearls Publishing; 2020. Available at: https://www.ncbi.nlm.nih.gov/books/NBK532895/.

11. Ginglen JG, Doyle MQ. Immunization. In: StatPearls [internet]. Treasure Island (FL): StatPearls Publishing; 2020. Available at: https://www.ncbi.nlm.nih.gov/books/NBK459331/.

12. Andre FE, Booy R, Bock HL, et al. Vaccination greatly reduces disease, disability, death and inequity worldwide. Bull World Health Organ 2008;86(2):81–160.

13. Healthy people 2020. Available at: https://www.healthypeople.gov/2020/topics-objectives/topic/immunization-and-infectious-diseases. Accessed December 28, 2020.

14. Pickering LK, Meissner HC, Orenstein WA, et al. Principles of vaccine licensure, approval, and recommendation for use. Mayo Clin Proc 2020;95(3):600–8.

15. Centers for Disease Control and Prevention. Immunization schedules. Recommended child and adolescent immunization schedule for ages 18 years or younger, United States, 2020. Available at: https://www.cdc.gov/vaccines/schedules/index.html. Accessed December 28, 2020.

16. Centers for Disease Control and Prevention. Immunization schedules. Recommended adult immunization schedule for ages 19 years or older, United States, 2020. Available at: https://www.cdc.gov/vaccines/schedules/index.html. Accessed December 28, 2020.

17. Centers for Disease Control and Prevention. Guidelines for vaccinating pregnant women. Available at: https://www.cdc.gov/vaccines/pregnancy/hcp-toolkit/guidelines.html. Accessed December 31, 2020.

18. Centers for Disease Control and Prevention. General best practice guidelines for immunization: best practice guidance of the advisory committee on immunization practices (ACIP). Available at: https://www.cdc.gov/vaccines/hcp/acip-recs/general-recs/special-situations.html. Accessed December 31, 2020.

19. Rubin LG, Levin MJ, Ljungman P, et al. 2013 IDSA clinical practice guideline for vaccination of the immunocompromised host. Clin Infect Dis 2014;58(3):309–18.

20. Thomson A, Robinson K, Vallée-Tourangeau G. The 5As: a practical taxonomy for the determinants of vaccine uptake. Vaccine 2016;34(8):1018–24.

21. Holman DM, Benard V, Roland KB, et al. Barriers to human papillomavirus vaccination among US adolescents: a systematic review of the literature. JAMA Pediatr 2014;168(1):76–82.

22. Ojinnaka CO, McClellan DA, Weston C, et al. Determinants of HPV vaccine awareness and healthcare providers' discussion of HPV vaccine among females. Prev Med Rep 2017;5:257–62.

23. Fazekas KI, Brewer NT, Smith JS. HPV vaccine acceptability in a rural southern area. Womens Health (Larchmt) 2008;17(4):539–48.

24. ED M, Janda J, JH E, et al. Vaccine hesitancy and refusal. J Pediatr 2016;175: 248–9.

25. Wakefield AJ, Murch SH, Anthony A, et al. RETRACTED: ileal-lymphoid-nodular hyperplasia, non-specific colitis, and pervasive developmental disorder in children. Lancet 1998;351(9103):637–41.

26. Gerber JS, Offit PA. Vaccines and autism: a tale of shifting hypotheses. Clin Infect Dis 2009;48(4):456–61.

27. Offit PA, Quarles J, Gerber MA, et al. Addressing parents' concerns: do multiple vaccines overwhelm or weaken the infant's immune system? Pediatrics 2002; 109(1):124–9.

28. McKenna KC. Use of aborted fetal tissue in vaccines and medical research obscures the value of all human life. Linacre Q 2018;85(1):13–7.

29. Krok-Schoen JL, Bernardo BM, Weier RC, et al. Belief about mandatory school vaccinations and vaccination refusal among ohio appalachian parents: do demographic and religious factors, general health, and political affiliation play a role? J Rural Health 2018;34(3):283–92.

30. Center for Disease Control. Exclusion of philosophical exemptions. Cal Health & Safety Code NH Code Admin R He-P 301. 2015;13(February):1-19. Available at: https://www.cdc.gov/phlp/docs/school-vaccinations.pdf. Accessed December 10, 2020.

31. National Conference of State Legislators. States with religious and philosophical exemptions from school immunization requirements. Available at: http://www.ncsl.org/research/health/school-immunization-exemption-state-laws.aspx. Accessed December 10, 2020.

32. Atwell JE, Van Otterloo J, Zipprich J, et al. Nonmedical vaccine exemptions and pertussis in California, 2010. Pediatrics 2013;132(4):624–30.

33. Brabin L, Roberts SA, Stretch R, et al. Uptake of first two doses of human papillomavirus vaccine by adolescent schoolgirls in manchester: prospective cohort study. BMJ 2008;336(7652):1056–8.

34. Smith LM, Kaufman JS, Strumpf EC, et al. Effect of human papillomavirus (HPV) vaccination on clinical indicators of sexual behaviour among adolescent girls: the Ontario Grade 8 HPV Vaccine Cohort Study. CMAJ 2015;187(2):E74–81.

35. Tanday S. HPV vaccinations do not encourage risky sexual behaviour. Lancet Oncol 2014;15(3):e109.

36. Prins W, Butcher E, Hall LL, et al. Improving adult immunization equity: where do the published research literature and existing resources lead? Vaccine 2017; 35(23):3020–5.

37. Washington HA. Medical apartheid: the dark history of medical experimentation on Black Americans from colonial times to the present LK - https://Butler.on. Worldcat.Org/Oclc/61131882. 1st ed. Doubleday; 2006. Available at: http://catdir.loc.gov/catdir/enhancements/fy0704/2005051873-s.html. Accessed September 15, 2020.

38. Grohskopf LA, Liburd LC, Redfield RR. Addressing Influenza Vaccination Disparities During the COVID-19 Pandemic. JAMA 2020;324(11):1029–30.

39. US Centers for Disease Control and Prevention. Coronavirus disease 2019 (COVID-19): health equity considerations and racial and ethnic minority groups.

Available at: https://www.cdc.gov/coronavirus/2019-ncov/community/health-equity/race-ethnicity.html. Accessed December 3, 2020.

40. Lu PJ, Rodriguez-Lainz A, O'Halloran A, et al. Adult vaccination disparities among foreign-born populations in the U.S., 2012. Am J Prev Med 2014;47(6): 722–33.

41. Reuben R, Aitken D, Freedman JL, et al. Mistrust of the medical profession and higher disgust sensitivity predict parental vaccine hesitancy. PLoS One 2020; 15(9):1–9.

42. Vyas D, Galal SM, Rogan EL, et al. Training students to address vaccine hesitancy and/or refusal. Am J Pharm Educ 2018;82(8):944–50.

43. Boom JA, Healy CM. Standard childhood vaccines: parental hesitancy or refusal. UpToDate 2020;1–26.

44. Pich J. Patient reminder and recall interventions to improve immunization rates: a cochrane review summary. Int J Nurs Stud 2019;91:144–5.

45. Kumar D, Noor N, Kashyap V. Vaccine hesitancy—issues and possible solutions. J Med Allied Sci 2018;8(2):55–8.

Health Disparities and Access to Care in the United States

Charles Regan, MS, PA-C*, Aimee Lamb, PA-C, MMSs,
Kenneth Early, CPNP-AC

KEYWORDS

- Healthcare disparities • Healthcare inequalities • Health inequities
- Social determinants of health • Access to care

KEY POINTS

- To define health care disparities.
- To understand the history and factors involved within the disparities.
- To identify risk factors within the ecological framework.
- To illustrate the differences and inequalities that exist.
- To demonstrate areas of improvement and weakness.

HISTORY

The history of health care disparities is not well known of its origin, which could be due to variations in terminology or lack of clear historical documentation. The concept that racial and ethnic minorities and the white majority have different health experiences has been well established (McKeown, Record, & Turner, 1975).[1] Disparities experienced by African Americans received significant national attention in 1985 when the US Department of Health and Human Services released the Report of the Secretary's Task Force on Black and Minority Health, also known as the Malone-Heckler report, which substantively documented racial and ethnic health disparities (Byrd & Clayton, 2000).[2] This remains to be an important time at which a growing concern into the reasons for the disparities sparked interest for further data collection and research; this is evidenced by a review into the term health disparities, which demonstrated that in their search of peer-reviewed literature, the term health disparities appear only once in the 1980s, 30 times in the 1990s, and in 4 hundred articles from 2000 to 2004 (Adler and Rehkopf, 2008).[3]

Physician Assistant Program, Department of Natural Sciences, College of Arts and Sciences, Lawrence Technological University, 21000 West Ten Mile Road, Southfield, MI 48075, USA
* Corresponding author.
E-mail address: cregan@ltu.edu

Physician Assist Clin 7 (2022) 141–147
https://doi.org/10.1016/j.cpha.2021.08.005
2405-7991/22/© 2021 Elsevier Inc. All rights reserved.
physicianassistant.theclinics.com

The goal of continuing to improve access to health care despite disparities remains to be a focus among researchers and health care professionals. To further explore disparities, we have to understand the concept of social determinants of health (SDOH) and its components. With that being said, there is no consensus on a single set of factors that define SDOH. However, it is helpful to review multiple frameworks that explore the SDOH. The WHO, Healthy People 2020, County Health Rankings Model 2014, and Kaiser Family Foundation 2018 all explore the makeup of these social determinants of health. If you look carefully in this figure, you will find that the Healthy People 2020 and Kaiser Family Foundation 2018 components are very similar with the separation of food environment from economic stability by the latter.

Access to health care has 4 components, each having an element of effect on access that is proposed by *Healthy People 2020* and they include coverage, services, workforce, and timeliness. Coverage becomes an issue for the uninsured or those not qualified who will have less health encounters that will directly result in poorer health. Services involve regular interval care and contain preventative practices that many individuals lack. Workforce consists of available well-qualified health care providers that are culturally competent. Timeliness involves being able to have the appropriate testing or services in the appropriate time frame, avoiding any unnecessary delays that can inadvertently affect the outcomes of the individual's health.

The workforce component can often be looked at as a barrier to health care. Diversity in the composition of the health care workforce is important because it affects outcomes, quality, safety, and satisfaction. Racial and ethnic concordance in health care provider-patient relationships has been shown to improve care. Race-concordant patient-provider relationships, as opposed to race-discordant, have been found to result in longer medical visits with higher ratings of positive affect, shared decision-making, and satisfaction (Schoenthaler, and colleagues, 2012).[4]

DEFINITION

Health care disparities are differences in access to or availability of medical facilities and services and variation in rates of disease occurrence and disabilities between population groups defined by socioeconomic characteristics such as age, ethnicity, economic resources, or gender and populations identified geographically (AHRQ, 2012).[5] There are little differences noted in the meaning or definition of the following other than the terms used when discussing health disparities, health inequalities, or health inequity. In fact, the terms are used interchangeably, whereas in the United States we use the term health disparities and in Europe the term health inequalities is used.

Another definition of health disparity is that used by the US Department of Health and Human Services, which is by all means not short and sweet but inclusively states, "any health-related factor—disease burden, diagnosis, response to treatment, quality of life, health behaviors and access to care, to name only a few—that exist among population groups. Health disparities are associated with a broad, complex, and interrelated array of factors, and may reflect: age, race, ethnicity, socioeconomic status, disability status, identity and expression (e.g., gender, racial, ethnic), geographic location (e.g., rural or urban environment), education, health care (e.g., access, quality), culture (e.g., norms, traditions, collective responses), health behaviors (e.g., smoking, violence, substance abuse), biological (e.g., sex, chronic inflammation, telomere attrition, cellular senescence) ... or a combination of these."

AGE

There exists a reason for age to be a factor, and most of the information out there looks at the elderly or geriatric patient having a potential for disparity, and with an average aging population usually resulting in increased functional impairment/limited mobility, which in itself will create less activity and increase risk factors for additional health conditions and diseases, it is no surprise to see why. But there is also the potential for infants and very young children to be another age group at risk due to limits of this age group needing regular provider office visits, immunizations, and monitoring of growth. If the parents of this age have any factors that limit their access to care (transportation, illness, and so forth) this indirectly burdens the infant/child. This article, however, focuses on the aging/elderly special group.

To address the contribution of these factors to health disparities related to aging, National Institutes of Aging (NIA) has supported research, for example, that found Alzheimer disease to be more prevalent among African Americans and Hispanics than among other ethnic groups in the United States. Other studies have found that lower socioeconomic status is associated with poorer health and reduced life-span in the United States. Scientists have also observed sex differences in health and longevity. For example, overall women live longer than men but are more likely to develop osteoporosis or depressive symptoms or to report functional limitations as they age; men, on the other hand, are more likely to develop heart disease, cancer, or diabetes (NIA).[6]

DISABILITY

Disabilities can exist in many forms but essentially have 2 entities with either being physical or mental. There are a variety of conditions that can cause either mental or physical disability. There is a direct impact on an individual's condition that could result in further decline in health related to disability. Not to mention the stigma associated with mental health and lack of accessing appropriate care to those who suffer mental health illnesses and conditions.

Anyone can become disabled at any time during his or her life span, said Haver-camp, and today, about 22% of adults and 14% of children in the United States are living with at least one disability, which includes any mental or physical trait that limits functional capacity. In fact, disabilities are so common that the World Health Organization has concluded that disability is a natural feature of the human condition (National Academies of Sciences, Engineering, and Medicine. 2018).[7]

There has been recent improvement regarding this scenario with advertisements and commercials that expose famous people requiring professional mental care. It is important now more than ever to be open and have discussions, and implementation of proper screenings, such as the Patient Health Questionnaire-9 (**Fig. 1**), often used during routine health care visits, can open the door to these kinds of discussions and identify those who need help.

SOCIOECONOMIC STATUS, RACE, AND ETHNICITY

It is difficult to separate socioeconomic status, race, and ethnicity in terms of health care disparities. Looking at access more specifically, major issues of disparity occur for poor people and Hispanics, with lesser but important issues for Blacks, American Indians, and Asians. Poor people have worse access to care than high-income people for all 8 core report measures. Hispanics have worse access for 88% of the core report measures, whereas Blacks and American Indians have worse access on half of the

NAME:_____   DATE:_____

Over the last 2 weeks, how often have you been
bothered by any of the following problems?
(use "✓" to indicate your answer)

	Not at all	Several days	More than half the days	Nearly every day
1. Little interest or pleasure in doing things	0	1	2	3
2. Feeling down, depressed, or hopeless	0	1	2	3
3. Trouble falling or staying asleep, or sleeping too much	0	1	2	3
4. Feeling tired or having little energy	0	1	2	3
5. Poor appetite or overeating	0	1	2	3
6. Feeling bad about yourself—or that you are a failure or have let yourself or your family down	0	1	2	3
7. Trouble concentrating on things, such as reading the newspaper or watching television	0	1	2	3
8. Moving or speaking so slowly that other people could have noticed. Or the opposite — being so figety or restless that you have been moving around a lot more than usual	0	1	2	3
9. Thoughts that you would be better off dead, or of hurting yourself	0	1	2	3

add columns   ____ + ____ + ____

(Healthcare professional: For interpretation of TOTAL,   TOTAL ____
please refer to accompanying scoring card).

10. If you checked off any problems, how difficult have these problems made it for you to do your work, take care of things at home, or get along with other people?	Not difficult at all ____
	Somewhat difficult ____
	Very difficult ____
	Extremely difficult ____

Fig. 1. Example of the PHQ-9 questionnaire that was developed by Pfizer, Inc. 1999.

measures. Asian Americans have worse access on 43% of the measures (Kronenfeld, 2013).[8] Multiple studies have documented that a common barrier facing minority populations is the ability to access both prevention-based and primary care health services (AHRQ, 2012).[5]

Data collected from 1950 to 1998 depict significantly higher rates of morbidity and mortality among African Americans in the United States. Also, note that coinciding with this are the comorbidities with increasing frequency among African Americans as well.

Racial and ethnic disparities in health care emerge from a historic context in which health care has been differentially allocated based on social class, race, and ethnicity. Unfortunately, despite public laws and sentiment to the contrary, vestiges of this history remain and negatively affect the current context of health care delivery. And despite the considerable economic, social, and political progress of racial and ethnic minorities, evidence of racism and discrimination remain in many sectors of American life (Smedley, 2002).[9]

We have come a long way, and there continues to be small strides of improvement with recent initiatives among many organizations to promote diversity, inclusion, and equity. These initiatives help to promote, celebrate, and expose the differences of genders, cultures, races, sexual orientations, and ethnicities. It will continue to be an important focus to identify and eliminate any barriers that get in the way of fair treatment, access, advancements, and opportunities.

GENDER IDENTITY AND SEXUAL ORIENTATION

Disparities based on gender identity and sexual orientation have been present in many ways including, but not limited to, health status, health coverage, and health behaviors. Literature reviews in public health, medicine, and nursing note a dearth of studies relating to lesbian, gay, bisexual, and transgender population and report a disproportionate focus on human immunodeficiency virus/AIDS and other sexually transmitted diseases (Boehmer, 2002; Snyder, 2011; Johnson, Smyer, and Yucha, 2012).[10–12]

Access to health insurance is a key area in which many same-sex couples face disadvantages due to barriers either by employer-sponsored health insurance or by the state in which they reside possibly not recognizing same-sex marriages, making them potentially ineligible for health care coverage by policies in place. Healthy People 2020 goals, set by the US federal government to monitor improvements in population health, now include improving "the health, safety, and well-being of lesbian, gay, bisexual, and transgender individuals" (US Department of Health and Human Services, 2010).[13]

GEOGRAPHIC LOCATION

The area in which a person lives can put them at an advantage or disadvantage depending on the location of the city, town, or village and whether they meet their

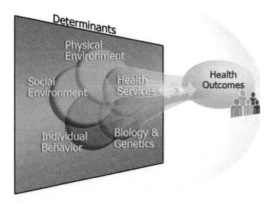

Fig. 2. Healthy People 2020. (Source: U.S. Department of Health and Human Services.)

criteria for urban or rural or the medically underserved due to lack of specific resources available or possible outcomes related to lack of availability. The US Department of Health and Human Services designates an area or population as medically underserved if having any of the following: too few primary care providers, high infant mortality, high poverty, or a high elderly population. Health Professional Shortage Areas are designated by Health Resources and Services Administration as having shortages of primary medical care, dental or mental health providers and may be geographic (a county or service area), population (eg, low income or Medicaid eligible) or facilities (eg, federally qualified health center or other state or federal prisons).[14]

SUMMARY

In conclusion, there are many factors that influence health care disparities. The World Health Organization in collaboration with the US Department of Health and Human Services provided a framework for the Healthy *People 2020*, which attempts to address the multiple factors by listing goals, mission, and a vision to create "a society in which all people live long, healthy lives." To truly address the health care disparities is to also improve the social determinants of health, which have a direct effect on better healthier outcomes. It will continue to be important to create awareness and recognition as well as continue data collection and research of health care disparities and access to care (**Fig. 2**) to monitor progress and identify areas needing improvement.

CLINICS CARE POINTS

- Identify potential negative SDOH in every patient by extrapolating thorough patient-centered histories.
- Once a negative SDOH has been identified, develop patient care that focuses to eliminate any disparity for better health outcomes.
- Evaluate trends within patient populations to help improve population health.
- Create diverse cultural competent evidence-based care that is accessible and affordable to all patients.

DISCLOSURE

The authors have nothing to disclose.

REFERENCES

1. McKeown T, Record RG, Turner RD. An interpretation of the decline of mortality in England and Wales during the twentieth century. Popul Stud 1975;29: 391–422.
2. Byrd WM, Clayton LA. An American health dilemma. In: Byrd WM, Clayton LA, editors. A medical history of African Americans and the problem of race: beginnings to 1900, vol. 1. New York: Routledge; 2000.
3. Adler NE, Rehkopf DH. U.S. Disparities in health: descriptions, causes, and mechanisms. Introduction. 2008. Available at: https://www.annualreviews.org/doi/abs/10.1146/annurev.publhealth.29.020907.090852. Accessed April 16, 2021.

4. Schoenthaler A, Chaplin WF, Allegrante JP, et al. Provider communication effects medication adherence in hypertensive African Americans. Patient Educ Couns 2009;75(2):185–91.
5. Agency for healthcare research and quality. Disparities. AHRQ. 2012. Available at: https://www.ahrq.gov/topics/disparities.html. Accessed April 16, 2021.
6. National Institute on Aging. U.S. Department of Health and Human Services. Goal F: Understand health disparities related to aging and develop strategies to improve the health status of older adults in diverse populations. Available at: https://www.nia.nih.gov/about/aging-strategic-directions-research/goal-health-disparities-adults#f1. Accessed April 15, 2021.
7. People living with disabilities: health equity, health disparities, and health literacy: proceedings of a workshop. The National Academies of Sciences, Engineering, and Medicine; 2018. Available at: https://www.ncbi.nlm.nih.gov/books/NBK526280/. Accessed April 16, 2021.
8. Kronenfeld JJ. Social determinants, health disparities and linkages to health and health care. In: Research in the sociology of health care, vol. 31. Emerald Publishing Group Ltd; 2013. p. 7.
9. Smedley BD, Stith AY. Committee on understanding and eliminating racial and ethnic disparities in health care. Unequal treatment: confronting racial and ethnic disparities in health care. National Academies Press; 2002.
10. Boehmer U. Twenty years of public health research: inclusion of lesbian, gay, bisexual, and transgender populations. Am J Public Health 2002;92(7):1125–30.
11. Snyder JE. Trend analysis of medical publications about LGBT persons: 1950-2007. J Homosex 2011;58(2):164–88.
12. Johnson M, Smyer T, Yucha C. Methodological quality of quantitative lesbian, gay, bisexual, and transgender nursing research from 2000 to 2010. ANS Adv Nurs Sci 2012;35(2):154–65.
13. United States Department of Health and Human Services. Healthy people goals 2020. Topic Areas. 2010. Available at: https://www.cdc.gov/nchs/healthy_people/hp2020/hp2020_topic_areas.htm. Accessed April 16, 2021.
14. MUA find. Health resources and service administration. Available at: https://data.hrsa.gov/tools/shortage-area/mua-find#:~:text=Medically%20Underserved%20Areas%2FPopulations%20are,or%20a%20high%20elderly%20population. Accessed April 16, 2021.

The Challenges of Providing Preventive Health Care in Rural America

DeShana Collett, PA-C, PhD[a], Kay Miller Temple, MD, MMC[b],*,
Roger D. Wells, PA-C[c]

KEYWORDS

- Rural health care • Access to care • Rural workforce • Social determinants of health
- Population health

KEY POINTS

- Rural health services and government demographic research find that rural populations are older, sicker, poorer, and have less access to education and health care.
- Health care access and health prevention activities for rural residents are intimately tied to their ability to access health care.
- The rural workforce concentration in primary care and medical specialties has significant on disease prevalence and prevention.
- There are social determinates of health that are unique to rural communities, making them more vulnerable to health care disparities and thus to health disparities.

INTRODUCTION

Rural America is routinely described in terms of a residual: that which is not urban. According to the US Census Bureau, nearly 20% of the population—about 60 million people—live on slightly more than 95% of the landmass.[1] Yet the contributions made by rural Americans that impact the other 80% of Americans' overall viability and health are manifold: food, energy, and recreation. Rural areas are also important to national security, with nearly 40% of the military members coming from rural areas.[2,3]

Definitions associated with rural demographics are many. Rural researchers suggest that the use of these multiple definitions, as required by federal, state, local agencies, and data resources may lead to confusion and inequity in the distribution of resources depending on the description used.[4]

[a] Department of Physician Assistant Studies, University of Kentucky College of Health Sciences, Room 205C Wethington Building, 900 South Limestone Street, Lexington, KY 40536, USA; [b] Rural Health Information Hub, Center for Rural Health, University of North Dakota School of Medicine and Health Sciences, 1300 North Columbia Road, Grand Forks, ND 58203, USA; [c] Lexington Regional Health Center, PO Box 980, 1201 North Erie, Lexington, NE 68850, USA
* Corresponding author.
E-mail address: kay.millertemple@und.edu

Physician Assist Clin 7 (2022) 149–165
https://doi.org/10.1016/j.cpha.2021.08.006
2405-7991/22/© 2021 Elsevier Inc. All rights reserved.
physicianassistant.theclinics.com

Definition controversies aside, rural health services and government demographic research find that rural populations are older, sicker, and poorer, and have less access to education and health care. Often thought only to be engaged in agriculture and livestock production, rural residents are also involved in mining, energy extraction, and manufacturing (**Fig. 1**).[5–7] The use of a racial and ethnic research lens reveals characteristics often overlooked: a rural demographic that is increasingly ethnically diverse[8] and an emerging younger population unable to access health care because of cost.[9]

Although similarities exist with inner-city populations, when these rural descriptors and characteristics are considered as a whole, they suggest a separate culture of health exists in rural America.[10] Recent publications provide insight into this latter possibility. Researchers based at the University of Kansas School of Social Welfare[11] noted 6 cultural characteristics, including a strong sense of independence and a strong connection to land or place (**Box 1**).

Part of these characteristics of culture include how rural residents themselves define health. A systematic literature review conducted by Gessert and colleagues[12] found consistent themes among rural populations that suggested that these populations tend to emphasize more functional aspects of health, like preservation of the ability to work and being able to continue in traditional social roles. Additionally, rural people tend to frame health in terms of independence and self-sufficiency, accepting ill-health with higher degrees of stoicism and seemingly more fatalism.[12] In summary, the context for the rural health landscape is as expressed by 1 rural health expert: Rural areas are resource restricted, but relationship rich.[13]

This article outlines how health care access barriers and rural-specific social determinants of health (SDOH) impact rural population disease prevention and the overall health and well-being of individuals living in rural America.

HEALTH CARE ACCESS

Health prevention activities for rural residents are intimately tied to their ability to access health care. An early definition of health care access came from a 1993 National Academy of Medicine report: the timely use of personal health care services to achieve the best health outcomes.[14] The Office of Disease Prevention and Health Promotion further elaborated that health care access requires 3 steps: gaining entry to a health care system, usually through insurance coverage; accessing the health care system, which implies a geographic availability tied to transportation; and finding a trusted

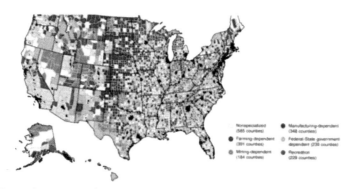

Fig. 1. Industry dependence for rural counties, 2010 to 2012. United States Department of Agriculture Economic Research Service Economic Information Bulletin 162. Rural America At A Glance. November 2016.

| **Box 1** |
| **Rural culture characteristics (2002–2009)** |
| Importance of family |
| Strong sense of independence |
| Connection to land or place |
| Conservatism |
| Influence of faith |
| Use of informal networks |
| *Adapted from* sources in Holmes, C. & Levy, M. University of Kansas School of Social Welfare. August 2015. This work was supported by a grant from the REACH Healthcare Foundation https://reachhealth.org/reports-publications/ |

provider with whom to establish a personal relationship.[15] Although many of these same issues exist in underserved urban areas, resources within urban metropolitan boundaries are not only present, but more concentrated in contrast with rural areas of the country where not uncommonly, resources are just nonexistent. For example, transportation may be more problematic for rural people owing to decreased proximity and hazardous road conditions that may impact adequate access to health care. Additionally, studies that have focused on rural occupations and health care access found that those who held jobs in time-intense occupations, like agriculture, had perceptions that justified placing the livelihood of person and family over personal health.

Multiple studies, gray literature reports, and advocacy organization policy briefs document the unique rural challenges to health care access.[16–18] Yet, these challenges must be acknowledged when considering that the first step in preventive interventions is health care access, and that health care access depends on adequate insurance coverage. When examining insurance coverage, one study reported responses from more than 850 rural residents and found that, in comparison with urban residents who often have employer-based insurance (53%), only 38% of rural residents had work-based coverage.[19] Another 13% had state-funded insurance coverage, such as Medicaid. Other reports point out that, for those seeking marketplace insurance coverage, premiums are significantly higher for rural residents.[20] Research has also indicated that rural Americans are significantly underinsured,[21] meaning that insurance deductibles and out-of-pocket health care costs exceed 5% or 10% of total income.[22]

Therefore, a relationship exists between access and insurance coverage that can lead to rural health disparities. Using cancer screening to exemplify how this link between access and insurance coverage impacts prevention activities, multiple studies[23–28] show that rural provider shortages lead to less screening even for those with coverage. Less screening can mean that, when a cancer is diagnosed, it is often in a more severe and advanced stage.[29] Additionally, these studies highlight how a lower provider concentration in less populated rural areas leads to longer wait times for wellness visits, during which prevention is discussed; also, travel to locations with screening infrastructure such as mammography leads to unaffordable out-of-pocket costs.

Another barrier to disease prevention work in rural areas is parity access for behavioral health services. Suicide and substance use disorder rates—substance use disorder, which leads to additional harm from increased human immunodeficiency virus and hepatitis C infection rates—occur at higher rates in rural than urban areas.[30,31] More than 65% of rural Americans receive mental health care from a primary health care provider. If a behavioral health crisis occurs, law enforcement personnel are usually the first to respond as opposed to a trained provider.[32]

A lack of behavioral health access for rural youth is especially problematic. A recent report that addressed suicide issues and behavioral health access found that highly rural areas had fewer mental health facilities and fewer suicide prevention services when compared with those in more urban areas.[33] Other researchers studying rural challenges to behavioral health access in rural low-income areas note that there is a hesitance to obtain services housed in a brick-and-mortar building because of the stigma of having a vehicle recognized in the parking lot[34]; in other words, there is an inherent loss of confidentiality when communities are small and personal vehicle recognition is high.

Rural workforce concentration also impacts preventive care. Only about 10% of physicians live in rural areas where 20% of the population resides.[35] For nearly 2 decades, physician assistants (PAs) and advanced practice nurses have increasingly filled the care gap created by the physician shortage. According to a 2012 Agency for Healthcare Research and Quality report, nurse practitioners and PAs are more likely to work in rural areas than physicians (16% vs 11%). The report also indicated that nurse practitioners and PAs who have specialized in primary care are much more likely to work in rural areas (28% and 25%, respectively) (**Table 1**).[36]

Despite the research suggesting that PAs are 1 solution to alleviating the workforce shortage, their profession continues to struggle with federal regulations that restrict the PA scope of practice. Studies have demonstrated that, when rural practices used a shared model that included PAs and advanced practice nurses working with physicians, this strategy not only increased access to care, but also resulted in a greater number of patients with unmet needs having adequate access to a provider.[37] Having access to a provider can take many forms and extends beyond traditional face-to-face interactions.

How the broad and deep the influence of rural hospital closures impacts rural population health and disease prevention measures is beyond the scope of this article. However, a 2017 recap from the Rural Health Research Gateway notes that nearly 800,000 people have lost the system they depended on for health care. Consequently, they will likely experience an increase in emergency medical services costs and an increase in travel time and transportation costs to other health care services. The most vulnerable patients—for example, those with limited resources and those in need of obstetric care—are also likely to experience the greatest health disparity owing to those lost services.[38]

SOCIAL DETERMINANTS OF HEALTH

In addition to the impact of rural health care access linked to insurance coverage and provider concentration, one study found that those categories in combination with socioeconomic factors accounted for nearly 80% of the total variance in rural and urban mortality rates.[39] This finding points to the importance of looking at issues of rural health and well-being other than those strictly related to health care access as having a marked impact on health and well-being. Using the framework provided by the SDOH, multiple variables that impact overall physical and psychological health can be examined. The SDOH are defined as the conditions in the environment where people are born, live, learn, work, play, worship, and age that affect a wide range of health, functioning, and quality-of-life outcomes and risks. Healthy People 2030 provides further categorization of SDOH using 5 subdivisions: economic stability, neighborhood and built environment, social and community environment, and education access and quality, and also includes health care access and quality.[40]

Table 1
Geographic distribution of health care professionals, 2010

Geography	All Specialties			Primary Care					US Population
	Nurse Practitioner	PA	Physicians	Nurse Practitioner	PA	Family Physicians/ General Practitioners	General Internal Medicine	General Pediatrics	
Urban	84.4%	84.4%	89.0%	72.2%	75.1%	77.5%	89.8%	91.2%	80%
Large rural	8.9%	8.8%	7.1%	11.0%	11.7%	11.1%	6.7%	6.2%	10%
Small rural	3.9%	3.8%	2.6%	7.7%	6.9%	7.2%	2.4%	1.8%	5%
Remote rural/frontier	2.8%	3.0%	1.3%	9.1%	6.3%	4.2%	1.1%	0.8%	5%

The Distribution of the U.S. Primary Care Workforce. Content last reviewed July 2018. Agency for Healthcare Research and Quality, Rockville, MD. https://www.ahrq.gov/research/findings/factsheets/primary/pcwork3/index.html.

The SDOH framework underscores the multiple unique characteristics of rural communities that make them more vulnerable to health disparities, especially rural communities that are continually plagued with economic instability. Acknowledging poverty as having a direct impact on health and health care status, the US Department of Agriculture reported that, in 2017, the rural poverty rate was more than 16%, compared with nearly 13% in urban areas.[40,41] With regard to income, even though the gap between rural and urban populations' unemployment rate is decreasing, changes in earned wage and income are not.[42,43]

The physical environment is another determinant that impacts rural health. Although clear blue skies, clean streams, and vast, untouched natural landscapes are often used to characterize rural areas, rural population health is impacted by common adverse air and water quality issues. Exposure to air pollution generated from conditions seen with agricultural practices, the burning of fossil fuels, and the spraying pesticides can have long-term detrimental health consequences, resulting in an increase in the prevalence of asthma and cardiopulmonary disease.[44] Recent increases in the frequency and intensity of wildfires that usually start in remote rural areas are also prompting public health concerns because of the relationship of smoke particulates to both acute and delayed respiratory diseases, like asthma and chronic obstructive pulmonary disease.[45]

There are unclear and concerning links between rural residence and lung disease. A recent study revealed that the rate of chronic obstructive pulmonary disease is twice that in rural poor areas when just comparing rural with national rates. And with regard to smoking cigarettes, there was a significant rural link with chronic obstructive pulmonary disease associated with poverty in rural individuals who had never smoked.[46]

Safe drinking water is also a concern in many rural communities relying on well water or groundwater as a drinking water source. These water sources are not subject to federal regulation and are commonly found to harbor harmful contaminants.[47,48] Private well water may contain high levels of nitrates, which has been linked to colorectal cancer.[49]

Last, 2 more socioeconomic factors have an impact on rural health disparities: education and health behaviors. Given the link between educational achievement and the ability to understand and use health information, lower health literacy scores in rural areas have been explained not just by differences in education, but by age, sex, race, ethnicity, and income.[50] Additionally, health behaviors in rural areas also lead to disparities. A 2017 public health report looking at 5 specific health-related behaviors, namely, smoking, alcohol consumption, activity levels, food consumption, and sleep hygiene, found that, although the prevalence of at least 4 of the health-related behaviors was achieved by less than one-third of the US population, it was lowest in the more rural counties.[51]

TRANSPORTATION

Understanding how both health care access and SDOH heavily impact rural health and well-being must include an understanding of the impact of transportation on both of these determinants—getting to medical appointments—local and at a distance—accessing pharmacies, getting to school and school activities (primary and secondary), consistently getting to jobs, accessing food, attending financial and legal appointments, and connecting with friends and family, along with all descriptions of social activities impact rural people's health and well-being. As 1 rural researcher stated, living a full and healthy life requires more than showing up for health care appointments.[52] And—as with so many other disparities—rural residents again come up short with options for transportation.

Tracking transportation data to analyze rural needs is in itself difficult. For example, researchers discovered that although 82% of rural counties had some form of public transportation, collected data grossly overestimated actual service because it failed to reflect areas within a county that were entirely without transportation options, a situation especially true in counties in Western states.[53]

The condition of rural transportation infrastructure is also problematic. According to the US Department of Transportation, nearly 40% of county roads are inadequate for current travel and 38,000 rural bridges longer than 20 feet are structurally deficient.[54]

A recent study found that transportation barriers continued to shift the site of care from an office-based setting to the more costly emergency room setting, a result also previously reported.[55] Even though rurality could not be discerned in this study, the researchers felt that their most notable discovery was that, beyond any sociodemographic or other health characteristics, the strongest association for transportation-related delayed care was for those individuals with health-related mobility limitations. This finding suggested that those requiring the greatest mobility assistance—perhaps use of assistive devices and similar—have the least access to transportation in rural and urban areas alike and poor outcomes are linked directly to that disparity.[55]

RURAL POPULATION HEALTH AND THE 5 LEADING CAUSES OF DEATH

In 2017, the Centers for Disease Control and Prevention (CDC) published 13 rural-focused studies,[56] including a report[57] on the leading causes of death in America. The reports provided a granular look at data that provided further insight into the links between higher death rates and potentially excess deaths often associated with various rural societal, geographic, behavioral, and structural factors.[58]

The first report[57] revealed that, across the rural–urban continuum, the 5 diseases that claim the most urban lives also claim the most rural lives: heart disease, cancer, stroke, chronic lower respiratory diseases, and unintentional injuries. The second report[58] further examined the rural–urban disparity of these deaths through a prevention lens, finding that, compared with metropolitan areas, nonmetropolitan areas have higher age-adjusted death rates and greater percentages of potentially excess deaths from the 5 leading causes of death. Not only did the disparity consistently exist on a national level and across the 10 public health regions, but the magnitude of the disparity raised concern at federal, state, regional, and local levels. Two years later, the CDC issued a follow-up report.[59] This follow-up study also included an analysis of potentially excess deaths. Calculating excess deaths by subtracting the expected number of deaths from the observed number of deaths, using data from the 3 best-performing states as the benchmark for expected deaths, potentially excess deaths[60] are those considered to be potentially preventable.

Because the 2017 report had used a binary metropolitan and nonmetropolitan analysis that could have masked important differences in health equity between rural areas themselves—because rural Arizona is unlike rural Maine—the 2019 report also examined the leading causes of death using a 6-category urban–rural classification. The data analysis included national, regional, and state-level results. With this closer look at national results, the 2019 report again found increasing rural excess deaths for heart disease, unintentional injuries, and chronic lower respiratory diseases (**Fig. 2**). For stroke, a quadratic trend was noted (a decrease followed by an increase). For cancer, deaths were decreased. The highest death rate disparity between the most rural counties (noncore) and urban areas was associated with chronic lower respiratory disease,[57] 57% percent compared with 13%.

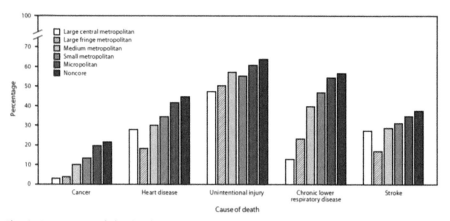

Fig. 2. Percentage of deaths that were potentially excess deaths among persons aged less than 80 years from the 5 leading causes of death, by urban–rural county classification—National Vital Statistics System, United States, 2017. (*From* Garcia MC, Rossen LM, Bastian B, et al. Potentially Excess Deaths from the Five Leading Causes of Death in Metropolitan and Nonmetropolitan Counties – United States, 2010-2017. MMWR Surveill Summ. 2019;68(10):1-11.)

On further examination of unintentional injuries included in the 2019 report, it is important to acknowledge that, decades ago, unintentional injuries were referred to as accidents.[61] Now these injuries are for the most part considered preventable.[61] At the state level in both urban and rural areas, unintentional injury deaths were increased, but in rural areas more slowly than urban. In rural areas, motor vehicle or transportation deaths are highest in number, followed by falls, with poisonings next, the latter of which notably includes opioid-related deaths. In urban areas, as opposed to the rural ranking, transportation and poisoning deaths are transposed.

Many factors influence rural transportation-related deaths. Distance to the treating facility may not always be a factor if the victims are dead on impact, as is often the case in rural areas. An examination of 2018 data showed that 67% of drivers killed in rural areas died at the scene, compared with 50% of drivers killed in urban areas.[62] Additionally, when comparing urban and rural drivers who died en route to hospitals, 58% were in rural and 41% in urban locations.

The results of these CDC analyses have spurred rurality inclusion in subsequent public health reports. The series has provided data for policymakers and advocacy organizations. For both urban and rural populations alike, the researchers noted that perhaps the most important limitation of the studies were that not all deaths are equally preventable among the leading causes, or within each leading cause. Noting the important differences in health equity between rural and urban areas in addition to differences between rural areas themselves—again, rural Arizona is unlike rural Maine—targeted improvement interventions may need to accommodate those differences because disease prevention interventions effective in urban areas may not be scalable to rural areas.

RURAL HEALTH DISPARITY SOLUTIONS

For the past 20 years, public health researchers and other analysts have been tracking rural health disparities. From all-cause mortality to maternal health to behavioral health disparities, a few disparity trajectories remain unchanged, but most are worsening.

The efforts of experts, advocates, and policymakers are currently operating with an eye toward stabilizing and shoring up the rural health care access sites in place while new transformative solutions are designed and tested.

Because the nation's health care system still centers around an individual purchasing their health care services, some rural residents benefited from the changes brought about by the 2010 Patient Protection and Affordable Care Act, mostly owing to Medicaid expansion. However, many rural residents did not fare as well. In a 2019 report,[63] marketplace data analysis demonstrated that the majority of the nonprofit insurance co-ops created by the new law went bankrupt as a result of the disappearance of contractual financial support offered through the risk corridor payments. The resulting insurance carrier gap left nearly 35% of rural counties with only 1 carrier.

For rural people purchasing coverage through nonmarketplace plans, premiums have increased by double digits along with increasing deductibles. However, the researchers emphasized that the risk corridor payments—which were expressly designed to induce participation in the new marketplace by decreasing the potential losses from inadequate predictability of costs—are still exactly the type of policy addition that is vital to the successful launch of a market-based program in a rural area.[63]

To help rural residents who are uninsured and underinsured, a rural safety net exists. In 2002, the National Advisory Committee on Rural Health & Human Services reported[64] on this rural network along with establishing a definition of the rural safety net:

A complex web of public and private professionals and institutions including public and or community hospitals, public health departments, Federally Qualified Health Centers, Rural Health Clinics, free clinics, and private providers that deliver a disproportionate share of health care and related services to the uninsured, underinsured, low-income, Medicare and Medicaid recipients. They provide this care because of legal requirements or out of a sense of charity and duty.

Through the decades, the rural safety network has experienced funding difficulties, yet its members continue to serve rural patients in need.[65]

In addition to the rural safety net brick-and-mortar health care facility sites where acute care and disease prevention interventions can occur, efforts to attract more health care providers to rural areas is on-going.[64] A unique rural approach is the successful grow-your-own programs that encourage rural residents to pursue health care training and return to a rural area for practice. Research has proved that, although this factor is the strongest predictor of choosing a rural practice, the number of health care professionals coming from these pipelines cannot solve the rural provider shortage issues.[66] Additional efforts include financial support in the form of loan repayment and scholarship programs at the federal, state, and local levels, along with similar efforts by various organizations with continued positive impact on shortages.[66] In recent years, federal support for increasing the number of graduate medical education rural training tracks includes the Rural Residency Planning and Development Program. Other examples are the Rural Training Collaborative, now a sustainable program that evolved from initial federal support. As mental health care gains parity with physical health care, behavioral health rural training tracks are also being developed.[67]

Additionally, new professional roles have been created to both help fill rural workforce gaps and to address access needs. For example, community health workers are emerging as health care professionals that add a different level of health care engagement as well as diversity to the rural workforce—diversity because they are only eligible for the position if they are members of the community they serve.[68] Defined by the American Public Health Association, a community health worker is a frontline public health worker who is a trusted member of and has an unusually close understanding of the community served. The relationship allows the worker to influence patient behaviors, facilitate access to services, and improve the quality and cultural competence of service delivery, further providing a positive impact in rural areas.[69]

Frequently used to address common medical conditions in urban America, in rural areas, community health workers are often trained as outreach generalists who can provide assessment services, disease prevention education, and other activities usually guided by the policies of the organizations employing the community health worker. In addition to providing education and addressing many aspects of health and well-being including the SDOH, one of the important ways community health workers provide disease prevention in rural areas is by instructing patients in chronic disease self-management programs.[70] The model used by the community health worker profession has shown not only to be more than popular with the populations they serve, but have been proven to be effective within insurance models providing care for high-risk populations.[69]

TRANSFORMATIVE SOLUTIONS

Although continued efforts focus on access issues, demonstration projects exist that are exploring alternative ways of impacting the growing gap between rural and urban health disparities. According to the Rural Health Information Hub, a website dedicated to information dissemination, demonstration projects are used on a limited and controlled scale to test and measure the effect of potential changes before programs are launched nationwide.[71] More than 20 completed and current projects have shown that demonstration projects are especially important to scale rural health care solutions and illustrate how implementing a demonstration project is one way to find out whether a new model of providing health care will meet rural needs.

Several of these projects involve global budgeting approaches. Supported by the Centers for Medicare and Medicaid Services Innovation Center and the state's health department, the Pennsylvania Rural Health Model provides a constant monthly revenue to participating hospitals as they redesign their care delivery system to improve access and focus on providing quality care.[72] Another project, the Rural Integration Models for Parents and Children to Thrive (IMPACT) Demonstration,[73] uses the 2-generational approach to address several SDOH by intentionally linking services needed by both parents and children, an approach resulting in increased economic security along with improved physical and mental well-being.

Improving rural health by leveraging rural local public health departments has also been proposed, with researchers proposing 5 prescriptions ranging from adjusting the definition of rural to help standardize support for rural public health departments to creating a rural population-based prevention agenda.[74]

IMPACT OF COVID-19 ON RURAL HEALTH CARE TRANSFORMATION

Telehealth is another solution aimed at bridging the access gap by allowing increased access to urban-based specialty health care and effectively negating much of the financial cost associated with transportation. The 2020 coronavirus disease (COVID-19) pandemic and public health emergency has highlighted the utility of telehealth as a valuable tool to meet not just urgent health care access needs, but also to be positioned as a sustained health care access format. Federal waivers have been granted for the multiple reimbursement elements associated with providing both urban-based specialty care as well as for local care in rural areas. Especially valuable have been waivers that included reimbursement for phone-only appointments. This option allowed both rural patients and providers without audiovisual infrastructure to access care and provide care. The waivers also expanded the types of health care professionals allowed to furnish distant site services to include all those who are eligible to bill Medicare for their professional telehealth services.[75]

Although telehealth seems almost a panacea for rural health care delivery, challenges still exist for it to be leveraged as a transformative solution to health care delivery. Barriers that impact its efficiency and effectiveness include difficulties in provider licensure across state lines, payer reimbursement, and a lack of rural broadband infrastructure. Although Rural Health Clinics are receiving reimbursement for telehealth, this practice is limited to the duration of the current public health emergency and new legislation will be required for an extension after the pandemic.

In the rural setting, care via telehealth highlights other unique challenges. To function effectively, patients and facilities must have adequate broadband and Internet infrastructure to conduct telehealth care. A recent report indicated that 77% of small counties do not have infrastructure that meets the Federal Communication Commission broadband definition.[76] A 2019 journal editorial also pointed out that, although wireless cellular technology and cloud-based videoconferencing capacity are rendering the Federal Communication Commission broadband standard less relevant and providing increased access, telehealth still does not address health care access capacity issues caused by provider shortages.[77]

The COVID-19 pandemic is also accomplishing what years of advocacy and numerous publications and demonstration projects could not: illustrating the value of telehealth. Providing care by remote connection is quickly becoming a standard of care for many medical and behavioral health conditions.[78] As the crisis emphasized the vulnerabilities in the fee-for-service model and negative operating margins, payment models like global budgeting continue to emerge as a mechanism that provides a stable revenue stream allowing for uninterrupted rural health care delivery.[79]

With the current process of shifting the rural paradigm from piecemeal medical care to a more holistic approach to health, again the coronavirus pandemic has emerged as a major influence. It is likely an understatement that the COVID-19 public health emergency will stand as a pivotal disruptor to rural health care delivery, especially in terms of hospital closures, telehealth, and reimbursement mechanisms. Proof comes from information in the surge of academic publications that how the crisis has impacted rural health care organizations and professionals.[74–80]

SUMMARY

Providing disease prevention to the rural population of 60 million people is a task that must equal the magnitude of the ethnoracial and geographic diversity of that population. These activities must accommodate mountains, forests, prairies, and deserts that total 95% of the country's landmass and also must include every permutation of inclement weather.

The focus of the disease prevention challenges and opportunities unique to each rural community will need to be on the patient experience that provides health outcomes that narrow the rural–urban health disparity gap. Access to care must reign foremost, with the need to ensure "essential access to an essential provider." Paramount will be acknowledging the social reality in which the rural provider serves along with the need to increase collaboration between rural public health departments, mental health providers, physical health providers, and community-based services to address rural SDOH. Such needs may require policy mandates and regulations, but because of inherent diversity within rural populations and rural geography, there must be regulatory flexibility to meet local needs.

CLINICS CARE POINTS

- For the US population residing in rural areas, disease prevention depends on the population's ability to access health care.
- Lack of health care access for preventive services in rural American is linked to the lack of primary care providers and medical and surgical specialists located in rural areas.
- Providers organizing preventive care for rural patients should be aware of transportation limitations and high costs of distance travel to needed services, which are often located in urban areas.

DISCLOSURE

The authors have nothing to disclose.

REFERENCES

1. America counts: stories behind the numbers: one in five Americans live in rural areas. U.S. Census Bureau; 2017. Available at: https://www.census.gov/library/stories/2017/08/rural-america.html. Accessed December 1, 2020.
2. Kleykamp M. When a simple statistic isn't so simple: the story of rural enlistments. Veteran Scholars; 2017. Available at: https://veteranscholars.com/2017/04/11/when-a-simple-statistic-isnt-so-simple-the-story-of-rural-enlistments/. Accessed December 1, 2020.
3. Baccam L. Veterans returning to civilian life bring skill and talent to farm and ranch. USDA; 2017. Available at: https://www.usda.gov/media/blog/2016/11/10/veterans-returning-civilian-life-bring-skill-and-talent-farm-and-ranch. Accessed December 1, 2020.
4. Bennett KJ, Borders TF, Holmes GM, et al. What is rural? Challenges and implications of definitions that inadequately encompass rural people and places. Health Aff (Millwood) 2019;38(12):1985–92.
5. Micropolitan America. U.S. Census Bureau; 2019. Available at: https://www.census.gov/library/visualizations/2019/demo/micropolitan-america.html. Accessed December 1, 2020.
6. The 2014 update of the rural-urban chartbook. Rural health reform policy research center. 2014. Available at: https://ruralhealth.und.edu/projects/health-reform-policy-research-center/pdf/2014-rural-urban-chartbook-update.pdf. Accessed December 1, 2020.
7. Rural America at a glance. United States Department of Agriculture Economic Research Service Economic Information Bulletin 162. 2016. Available at: https://www.ers.usda.gov/webdocs/publications/80894/eib-162.pdf?v=4410.5. Accessed December 1, 2020.
8. Sharp G, Lee BA. New faces in rural places: patterns and sources of nonmetropolitan ethnoracial diversity since 1990. Rural Sociol 2017;82(3):411–43.
9. James CV, Moonesinghe R, Wilson-Frederick SM, et al. Racial/ethnic health disparities among rural adults - United States, 2012-2015. MMWR Surveill Summ 2017;66(23):1–9.
10. Thomas TL, DiClemente R, Snell S. Overcoming the triad of rural health disparities: how local culture, lack of economic opportunity, and geographic location instigate health disparities. Health Educ J 2014;73(3):285–94.
11. Holmes C, Levy M. Rural culture competency in health care white paper. University of Kansas School of Social Welfare; 2015. Available at: https://reachhealth.

org/wp-content/uploads/2016/12/REACH-RCC-White-Paper-Final.pdf. Accessed December 1, 2020.

12. Gessert C, Waring S, Bailey-Davis L, et al. Rural definition of health: a systematic literature review. BMC Public Health 2015;15:378.

13. Population health in rural America in 2020 – a virtual workshop. National Academies of Medicine; 2020. Available at: https://www.nationalacademies.org/event/06-24-2020/population-health-in-rural-america-in-2020-a-virtual-workshop. Accessed December 1, 2020.

14. Access to health care in America. Washington (DC): National Academies Press (US); 1993. 1, Introduction. Available at: https://www.ncbi.nlm.nih.gov/books/NBK235885/. Accessed December 1, 2020.

15. Office of Disease Prevention and Health Promotion. Healthy people 2020. Available at: https://www.healthypeople.gov/2020/topics-objectives/topic/Access-to-Health-Services. Accessed December 1, 2020.

16. Probst J, Eberth JM, Crouch E. Structural urbanism contributes to poorer health outcomes for rural America. Health Aff (Millwood) 2019;38(12):1976–84.

17. Healthcare Access in Rural Communities. Rural Health Information Hub, 2019. Healthcare Access in Rural Communities [online]. Rural Health Information Hub. Available at: https://www.ruralhealthinfo.org/topics/healthcare-access. Accessed December 1, 2020.

18. Challenges facing rural communities and the roadmap to ensure local access to high-quality, affordable care. American Hospital Association; 2019. Available at: https://www.aha.org/system/files/2019-02/rural-report-2019.pdf. Accessed December 1,2020.

19. Transamerica Center for Health Studies®. Left behind: health care in rural America. 2020. Available at:https://www.transamericacenterforhealthstudies.org/docs/default-source/fact-sheets/urbanicity/tchs-urbanicity-report_finald2d0c3eb2fff47e89c31d5c122e014b2.pdf. . Accessed December 1, 2020.

20. Robert Wood Johnson Foundation. Are marketplace premiums higher in rural than in urban areas?. 2018. Available at: https://www.rwjf.org/content/dam/farm/reports/issue_briefs/2018/rwjf449986. Accessed December 1, 2020.

21. Centers for Medicare and Medicaid Services. Rural health strategy. 2018. Available at: https://www.cms.gov/About-CMS/Agency-Information/OMH/Downloads/Rural-Strategy-2018.pdf. Accessed December 1, 2020.

22. Healthwell Foundation. Underinsured Americans need a financial lifeline 2015. Available at: https://www.healthwellfoundation.org/wp-content/uploads/2017/10/Underinsurance_In_America.HWF_.2015.pdf. Accessed December 1, 2020.

23. Doescher MP, Jackson JE. Trends in cervical and breast cancer screening practices among women in rural and urban areas of the United States. J Public Health Manag Pract 2009;15(3):200–9.

24. Carney PA, O'Malley J, Buckley DI, et al. Influence of health insurance coverage on breast, cervical, and colorectal cancer screening in rural primary care settings. Cancer 2012;118(24):6217–25.

25. Molina Y, Zimmermann K, Carnahan LR, et al. Rural women's perceptions about cancer disparities and contributing factors: a call to communication. J Cancer Educ 2018;33(4):749–56.

26. Bonafede MM, Miller JD, Pohlman SK, et al. Breast, cervical, and colorectal cancer screening: patterns among women with Medicaid and commercial insurance. Am J Prev Med 2019;57(3):394–402.

27. Orwat J, Caputo N, Key W, et al. Comparing rural and urban cervical and breast cancer screening rates in a privately insured population. Soc Work Public Health 2017;32(5):311–23.

28. Nfonsam VN, Vijayasekaran A, Pandit V, et al. Patients diagnosed with colorectal cancer in rural areas in Arizona typically present with higher stage disease. J Gastrointest Dig Syst 2015;5(5):346.

29. Zahnd WE, Fogleman AJ, Jenkins WD. Rural-Urban Disparities in Stage of Diagnosis Among Cancers With Preventive Opportunities. Am J Prev Med 2018;54(5):688–98.

30. Pettrone K, Curtin SC. Urban-rural differences in suicide rates, by sex and three leading methods: United States, 2000-2018. NCHS Data Brief 2020;(373):1–8.

31. Ali MM, Nye E, West K. Substance use disorder treatment, perceived need for treatment, and barriers to treatment among parenting women with substance use disorder in US rural counties. J Rural Health 2020. https://doi.org/10.1111/jrh.12488.

32. National Institute of Mental Health Office for Research on disparities and global mental health 2018 webinar series. Bethesda, MD. Available at: https://www.nimh.nih.gov/news/media/2018/mental-health-and-rural-america-challenges-and-opportunities.shtml. Accessed December 1, 2020.

33. Graves JM, Abshire DA, Mackelprang JL, et al. Association of rurality with availability of youth mental health facilities with suicide prevention services in the US. JAMA Netw Open 2020;3(10):e2021471.

34. Crumb L, Mingo TM, Crowe A. "Get over it and move on": the impact of mental illness stigma in rural, low-income United States populations. Ment Health Prev 2019;13:143–8.

35. Hing E, Hsiao CJ. State variability in supply of office-based primary care providers: United States, 2012. NCHS Data Brief 2014;(151):1–8.

36. Distribution of primary care workforce. Agency for Healthcare Research and Quality; 2012. Available at: https://www.ahrq.gov/sites/default/files/publications/files/pcwork3.pdf. Accessed December 1, 2020.

37. Xue Y, Goodwin JS, Adhikari D, et al. Trends in primary care provision to Medicare beneficiaries by physicians, nurse practitioners, or physician assistants: 2008-2014. J Prim Care Community Health 2017;8(4):256–63.

38. Schroder, S. Rural Health Research Recap. Effects of Rural Hospital Closures. Rural Health Research Gateway. Available at: https://www.ruralhealthresearch.org/assets/826-3293/effects-of-rural-hospital-closures-recap.pdf. Accessed December 1, 2020.

39. Gong G, Phillips SG, Hudson C, et al. Higher US rural mortality rates linked to socioeconomic status, physician shortages, and lack of health insurance. Health Aff 2019;38(12):2003–10.

40. Healthy people 2030, U.S. Department of Health and Human Services, Office of Disease Prevention and Health Promotion. Available at: https://health.gov/healthypeople/objectives-and-data/social-determinants-health. Assessed December 1, 2020.

41. Rural America at a glance 2018 edition. United States Department of Agriculture; 2018. Available at: https://www.ers.usda.gov/webdocs/publications/90556/eib-200.pdf. Assessed December 1, 2020.

42. Thiede BC, Lichter DT, Slack T. Working, but poor: the good life in rural America? J Rural Stud 2018;59:183–93.

43. Rural communities: age, income, and health status. Rural health research gateway. 2018. Available at: https://www.ruralhealthresearch.org/assets/2200-8536/rural-communities-age-income-health-status-recap.pdf. Accessed September 19,2020.

44. Manisalidis I, Stavropoulou E, Stavropoulos A, et al. Environmental and health impacts of air pollution: a review. Front Public Health 2020;8:14.

45. Liu JC, Wilson A, Mickley LJ, et al. Wildfire-specific fine particulate matter and risk of hospital admissions in urban and rural counties. Epidemiology 2017;28(1): 77–85.

46. Raju S, Keet CA, Paulin LM, et al. Rural residence and poverty are independent risk factors for chronic obstructive pulmonary disease in the United States. Am J Respir Crit Care Med 2019;199(8):961–9.

47. Lukens J. Running clear: preventing private water sources from becoming a health hazard in rural America. Rural Health Information Hub. 2019. Available at: https://www.ruralhealthinfo.org/rural-monitor/private-water-sources/. Accessed December 1, 2020.

48. Strosnider H, Kennedy C, Monti M, et al. Rural and urban differences in air quality, 2008-2012, and community drinking water quality, 2010-2015 - United States. MMWR Surveill Summ 2017;66(13):1–10.

49. Schullehner J, Hansen B, Thygesen M, et al. Nitrate in drinking water and colorectal cancer risk: a nationwide population-based cohort study. Int J Cancer 2018;143(1):73–9.

50. Zahnd WE, Scaife SL, Francis ML. Health literacy skills in rural and urban populations. Am J Health Behav 2009;33(5):550–7.

51. Matthews KA, Croft JB, Liu Y, et al. Health-related behaviors by urban-rural county classification - United States, 2013. MMWR Surveill Summ 2017; 66(5):1–8.

52. Henning-Smith C. The public health case for addressing transportation-related barriers to care. Am J Public Health 2020;110(6):763–4.

53. Mattson J. Rural transit fact book 2017. Small urban & rural transit center upper great plains transportation. Institute North Dakota State University; 2017. Available at: https://www.surtc.org/transitfactbook/downloads/2017-ruraltransit-factbook.pdf. Accessed December 1, 2020.

54. TIFIA rural project initiative. U.S. Department of Transportation; 2020. Available at: https://www.transportation.gov/buildamerica/financing/tifia/tifia-rural-project-initiative-rpi. Accessed December 1, 2020.

55. Wolfe MK, McDonald NC, Holmes GM. Transportation barriers to health care in the United States: findings from the National Health Interview Survey, 1997-2017. Am J Public Health 2020;110(6):815–22.

56. Centers for Disease Control and Prevention. Morbidity and mortality weekly report. MMWR rural health series. 2017. Available at: https://www.cdc.gov/mmwr/rural_health_series.html. Accessed December 1, 2020.

57. Moy E, Garcia MC, Bastian B, et al. Leading causes of death in nonmetropolitan and metropolitan areas- United States, 1999-2014 [published correction appears in MMWR Morb Mortal Wkly Rep. 2017 Jan 27;66(3):93]. MMWR Surveill Summ 2017;66(1):1–8.

58. Garcia MC, Faul M, Massetti G, et al. Reducing potentially excess deaths from the five leading causes of death in the rural United States [published correction appears in MMWR Morb Mortal Wkly Rep. 2017 Jan 27;66(3):93]. MMWR Surveill Summ 2017;66(2):1–7.

59. Garcia MC, Rossen LM, Bastian B, et al. Potentially excess deaths from the five leading causes of death in metropolitan and nonmetropolitan counties - United States, 2010-2017. MMWR Surveill Summ 2019;68(10):1–11.

60. Potentially Excess Deaths. National vital statistics system. National Center for Health Statistics; 2020. Available at: https://www.cdc.gov/nchs/nvss/potentially_excess_deaths.htm. Accessed December 1, 2020.

61. Temple KM. Rural Health Information Hub. Rural unintentional injuries: they're not accidents – they're preventable. Rural Health information Hub. 2017. Available at: https://www.ruralhealthinfo.org/rural-monitor/unintentional-injuries/. Accessed December 1, 2020.

62. Traffic safety facts. Rural/urban comparison of traffic fatalities 2018 data. National Highway Traffic Safety Administration. 2020. Available at: https://crashstats.nhtsa.dot.gov/Api/Public/ViewPublication/812957. Accessed December 1, 2020.

63. Barker AR, McBride TD, Mueller KJ, et al. The market mechanism and health insurance in rural places: lessons learned from an economics and policy perspective. RUPRI Center for Rural Health Policy Analysis University of Iowa, College of Public Health; 2019. Available at: https://rupri.public-health.uiowa.edu/publications/policypapers/Market%20Structures%20in%20Rural.pdf. Accessed December 1, 2020.

64. A targeted look at the rural health care safety net a report to the secretary, U.S. Department of Health and Human Services. National Advisory Committee on Rural Health & Human Services. 2002. Available at: https://www.hrsa.gov/sites/default/files/hrsa/advisory-committees/rural/reports-recommendations/2002-report-to-secretary.pdf. Accessed December 1, 2020.

65. Impact of COVID-19 on Rural Health Safety Net. The Chartis center for rural health. 2020. Available at: https://www.chartis.com/resources/files/CCRH_Research_Update-Covid-19.pdf. Accessed December 1, 2020.

66. MacQueen IT, Maggard-Gibbons M, Capra G, et al. Recruiting rural healthcare providers today: a systematic review of training program success and determinants of geographic choices. J Gen Intern Med 2018;33(2):191–9.

67. Guerrero APS, Balon R, Beresin EV, et al. Rural mental health training: an emerging imperative to address health disparities. Acad Psychiatry 2019;43(1):1–5.

68. Chaidez V, Palmer-Wackerly AL, Trout KE. Community health worker employer survey: perspectives on CHW workforce development in the Midwest. J Community Health 2018;43(6):1145–54.

69. Crespo R, Christiansen M, Tieman K, et al. An emerging model for community health worker-based chronic care management for patients with high health care costs in rural Appalachia. Prev Chronic Dis 2020;17:E13.

70. Anekwe TD, Rahkovsky I. Self-management: a comprehensive approach to management of chronic conditions. Am J Public Health 2018;108(Suppl 6):S430–6.

71. Tools for success. Testing new approaches. Rural health information hub. 2020. Available at: https://www.ruralhealthinfo.org/new-approaches. Accessed December 1, 2020.

72. The Pennsylvania rural health model. Centers for Medicaid and Medicaid services innovation center. 2020. Available at: https://innovation.cms.gov/innovation-models/pa-rural-health-model. Accessed December 1, 2020.

73. Implementation of the federal rural IMPACT demonstration. Office of the assistant secretary for planning and evaluation. Department of Health and Human Services; 2016. Available at: https://aspe.hhs.gov/system/files/pdf/224826/ImplementationFederalRuralIMPACT.pdf. Accessed December 1, 2020.

74. Leider JP, Meit M, McCullough JM, et al. The state of rural public health: enduring needs in a new decade. Am J Public Health 2020;110(9):1283–90.

75. Physicians and other clinicians: CMS flexibilities to fight COVID-19. Centers for Medicare and Medicaid Services; 2020. Available at: https://www.cms.gov/files/document/covid-19-physicians-and-practitioners.pdf. Accessed December 1, 2020.
76. Understanding the true state of connectivity in America. National Association of Counties; 2020. Available at: https://www.naco.org/resources/featured/understanding-true-state-connectivity-america. Accessed December 1, 2020.
77. Struminger BB, Arora S. Leveraging telehealth to improve health care access in rural America: it takes more than bandwidth. Ann Intern Med 2019;171(5):376–7.
78. Uscher-Pines L, Thompson J, Taylor P, et al. Where virtual was already reality: the experiences of a nationwide telehealth service during the COVID-19 pandemic. J Med Internet Res 2020. https://doi.org/10.2196/22727.
79. Fried JE, Liebers DT, Roberts ET. Sustaining rural hospitals after COVID-19: the case for global budgets. JAMA 2020;324(2):137–8.
80. The Lancet Global Health. Publishing in the time of COVID-19. Lancet Glob Health 2020;8(7):e860.

Population Health - Policy level

Preventing and Treating Tobacco Use

Nicole Ferschke, MMS, MBS, PA-C

KEYWORDS

- Tobacco cessation • Smoking related cancer • Smoking related disease
- Nicotine dependence • Tobacco prevention • Nicotine replacement therapy
- Pharmacologic therapy for smoking cessation
- Nonpharmacologic therapy for smoking cessation

KEY POINTS

- Tobacco use is a common problem associated with significant cost, morbidity, and mortality.
- Prevention measures are often targeted at preventing youth from initiating tobacco use.
- Patients need to be screening regularly for tobacco use and willingness to quit.
- Clinicians can use a number of pharmacologic and nonpharmacologic treatments, often in combination to help patients stop smoking.

INTRODUCTION

Although the use of tobacco products has declined over the past 50 years, smoking continues to be the leading cause of preventable death in the United States.[1] Chronic health conditions related to tobacco use accounted for $170 billion in health care dollars spent in the United States per year from 2006 to 2010 and cause more than 400,000 deaths per year.[2,3] As recently as 2019, an approximate 34.1 million US adults reported being current smokers, which is roughly 14% of the adult population.[3] Moreover, smokers are now using more than 1 tobacco product, including cigarettes, cigars, e-cigarettes, hookah, and smokeless tobacco.[1,4] This factor creates a rapidly evolving problem that health care providers must contend with while continuing to give patients the best prevention and cessation information possible.

Large disparities in tobacco use exist across many groups.[1] Smokers are more likely to be male. Native Americans have a higher prevalence of tobacco use than any other ethnic or racial group in the United States. Additionally, current and former military, members of LGBT+ groups, people with mental illness, and the disabled are more likely to use tobacco. Those without a high school education or who have a GED

Department of Physician Assistant Studies, Northern Arizona University, Phoenix Biomedical Campus, 435 North 5th Street, Phoenix, AZ 85004, USA
E-mail address: nicole.ferschke@nau.edu

Physician Assist Clin 7 (2022) 167–179
https://doi.org/10.1016/j.cpha.2021.08.007
2405-7991/22/© 2021 Elsevier Inc. All rights reserved.

and those who come from lower socioeconomic status (annual income of <$35,000 per year) have higher rates of tobacco use.[3]

The Population Assessment of Tobacco and Health (PATH) study, published in 2014, used data from more than 45,000 participants in the United States aged 12 and over.[4] The PATH study found that 28% of adults surveyed (aged $\geq$25 years) were current tobacco users and use of multiple tobacco products was reported in approximately 40% of respondents. The use of cigarettes was most common, followed by cigars, e-cigarettes, hookah, and smokeless tobacco. Men were more likely to use any tobacco product as compared with women (34.8% vs 20.8%, respectively). Other significant demographic characteristics included higher incidences among racial minorities, members of sexual minorities, lower education levels, lower household income, and those living in the South or Midwest United States. These findings are similar to other national surveys, including the National Survey on Drug Use and Health and the National Adult Tobacco Survey.[5,6] A summary of these surveys can be found in **Table 1**.

The 2017 National Health Interview Survey estimated that 47.7 million US adults (19.3%) currently used any tobacco product, and reported similar demographic characteristics with higher prevalence of tobacco use as seen in the PATH study.[7] Differences in incidence of tobacco use between these aforementioned sources likely stem from multiple factors. First, data were collected 3 years apart, and the lower numbers in the National Health Interview Survey could represent continued declines in tobacco use. Additionally, the PATH study surveyed just more than 45,000 persons 12 year of age and older, whereas the National Health Interview Survey was a population estimate based on a survey of approximately 26,000 adults. Regardless, these sources show that tobacco use is a persistent problem among American adults that disproportionately affects certain demographic groups.

HEALTH IMPACT OF TOBACCO USE

Tobacco use affects far more than the respiratory system. Smokers are at higher risk for a multitude of diseases and smoking is associated with an increase in all-cause mortality.[1] Smoking causes inflammation and impairs function of the immune system. Additionally, smokers must cope with the challenges of physiologic and physical dependence on nicotine.[8] Tobacco use is associated with billions of dollars spent aside from health care–related costs; this amount includes the cost of the products paid by the consumer, as well as money spent by the tobacco industry in advertising, and costs that result from lost productivity associated with tobacco-related illness and secondhand smoke exposure.[9] Exposure to secondhand smoke has been shown to be linked to cancer and respiratory and cardiovascular diseases, as well as leading to adverse health effects of the developing fetus, infants, and children.[1]

Tobacco use continues to be a significant modifiable risk factor for disease and death.[1] Smoking increases risk for a multitude of cancers, as well as diseases of the cardiovascular system, cerebrovascular disease, peripheral vascular disease, and chronic lung disease. Smoking can lead to pregnancy complications and cause illness and disease in those who are exposed to secondhand smoke. Additionally, studies have shown that smokers are at increased morbidity and mortality for multiple disease states not believed to have direct association to smoking, but smokers have poorer prognoses. Last, it is important to take into consideration the physiologic and psychological dependence to nicotine that smokers contend with, because this is the predominant reason why smokers ultimately have such difficulty with cessation.[10]

Table 1
Results of national tobacco surveys 2014

Survey	Incidence of Use in Adults	Incidence of Use in Youth	Product Used
Population Assessment of Tobacco and Health 2013–2014, n = 45,971	38% of 18- to 24-year-olds >25% of adults >25 years old	3% of 12- to 14-year-olds 15% of 15- to 17-year-olds	Cigarette use most prevalent 40% used more than one product (cigarettes plus e-cigarettes most common)
National Survey on Drug Use and Health 2014, n = 67,901	35% of 18- to 25-year-olds 25.9% adults over 26	7% of 12- to 17-year-olds	Results reported of any tobacco use
National Adult Tobacco Survey 2013–2014, n = 75,233	21.3% of adults (18 and over)	Not surveyed	Results reports of any tobacco use

Data from Refs.[4–6]

Smoking-Related Cancers

Much has been learned about the harms of cigarette smoking since the 1964 US Surgeon General's Advisory Committee Report concluded that cigarette smoking causes lung cancer.[11] Cigarette smoke contains at least 60 known carcinogens, and smoking accounts for at least 30% of all cancer-related deaths.[1,12] Smoking is the primary risk factor for 80% of lung cancer deaths and is the leading cause of cancer death in both men and women. Additionally, smoking increases the risk of developing up to 18 types of cancers, listed in **Box 1**, and worsens cancer outcomes, not only in cancers associated with smoking, but also in patients with breast, prostate, and other cancers.[12] Smoking is also associated with developing secondary malignancies, as well as increased all-cause mortality and cancer-specific mortality.[1]

Smoking-Related Disease

In addition to lung cancer, tobacco use is associated with multiple chronic diseases of the respiratory system; furthermore, smokers are at increased risk for respiratory infections. Smoking is the primary cause in 80% of cases of chronic obstructive pulmonary disease.[1] Mortality from chronic obstructive pulmonary disease has increased dramatically since the 1960s. Smoking (both in smokers and owing to secondhand exposure) is linked to an increased incidence of asthma in adolescents and adults and related to asthma exacerbations in all ages. Smoking is a major cause of cardiovascular disease (CVD) and is an attributing factor to 1 in 4 deaths owing to CVD.[1] Smoking remains a modifiable risk factor for several types of CVD, including atherosclerosis, coronary heart disease, stroke, peripheral vascular disease, and abdominal aortic aneurysm.

Studies have shown a relationship between the inflammatory process and oxidative stress created by smoking to the development of type 2 diabetes mellitus.[1] Smokers are at a 30% to 40% higher risk of developing type 2 diabetes mellitus than those who were never smokers, a risk that increases with the number of cigarettes smoked per day. Additionally, studies have shown that nicotine may cause insulin resistance.

Box 1
Cancers with known associations to smoking

- Lung
- Head and neck
- Leukemia
- Esophagus
- Bladder
- Pancreas
- Kidney
- Liver
- Stomach
- Colorectal
- Cervix
- Uterus
- Ovaries

Data from Ref.[12]

Smokers with diabetes are more likely to develop CVD, renal disease, peripheral vascular disease, retinopathy, and peripheral neuropathy.

Nicotine Dependence

Cigarette smoking was once thought to be a habit of personal choice; however, it is now known that nicotine addiction is the primary drive for the continuation of this behavior.[10] In addition to physiologic dependence, the act of smoking is a deeply ingrained learned behavior.[8] Nicotine is a highly addictive substance; the nicotine contained in cigarette smoke is absorbed from the lungs delivered rapidly (within 10–16 seconds), where it enters the bloodstream and travels to the brain. [10] The half-life of nicotine is 15 to 20 minutes, with a terminal half-life of approximately 2 hours. Smokers experience repetitive and transient high blood nicotine levels after each cigarette, and many smokers need hourly cigarettes to maintain nicotine concentrations. Overnight, nicotine levels can reach that of a nonsmoker; smokers report the first cigarette of the day the most satisfying, largely because symptoms of nicotine withdrawal are already beginning. Ultimately, this nicotine dependence is the primary reason why many smokers fail at cessation attempts.

TOBACCO USE PREVENTION STRATEGIES

Tobacco use prevention campaigns are largely aimed at youth, specifically adolescents. Eighty-six percent of adult daily smokers tried tobacco products before the age of 18.[1] Tobacco control measures have been shown to be effective at decreasing tobacco use. Adolescents and young adults are more likely to be impulsive and may demonstrate higher risk-taking behavior.[13] Young people who have friends who smoke, as well as those from lower socioeconomic status, are more likely to have earlier initiation of tobacco use.[13,14]

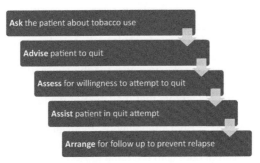

Fig. 1. The 5 *As* model for brief intervention. (*Adapted from* Ref.[19])

Limiting exposure to tobacco product advertising can be used as a tobacco use prevention strategy. Adolescent exposure to tobacco marketing has been shown previously to be associated with the initiation and continuation of tobacco use.[14,15] Additionally, African American and Hispanic individuals are more likely to report exposure to tobacco marketing.[16] Most exposures to tobacco marketing occur at stores, particularly convenience stores and gas stations.[16,17] Increased exposure to tobacco marketing has been found to be associated with more favorable attitudes toward the marketing and a higher likelihood of tobacco use.[17]

Product regulation has the potential to contribute to risk reduction. Increased prices of tobacco products from taxes help to prevent the initiation of use and promote cessation.[18] Legislation has been crucial to improving health outcomes and preventing use by creating smoke-free environments. Increasing the minimum age of purchase to 21 years is associated with lower smoking rates in youth and young adults.[1,8]

TOBACCO USE CESSATION STRATEGIES

Numerous cessation strategies are available to help smokers quit.[19] More than 70% of smokers visit a clinician yearly, and most report wanting to stop smoking. It is the responsibility of the clinician to assess every patient for tobacco use and ascertain if they wish to quit. Tobacco use should be seen as a chronic disease that requires repeated assessment and intervention. Smokers are more likely to be successful in cessation attempts when combinations of pharmacologic and nonpharmacologic options are used.

Most states have added at least partial Medicaid coverage for tobacco cessation treatment, as do Medicare, the Veteran's Health Administration, and the US military.[2,19] Making tobacco dependence a covered benefit increases the likelihood of successful cessation treatment. Additionally, every US state has telephone quit lines available, which can be beneficial to those smokers whose coverage does not include tobacco cessation counseling.

The initial intervention in this process is to first screen for tobacco use, then to determine whether the patient is willing to quit.[19] Once these patients are identified, the clinician can identify the most appropriate treatment. Using a brief intervention during the course of every patient encounter can significantly increase cessation rates, as well as prevent relapse. The 5 *As* model, outlined in **Fig. 1**, is one method a clinician can use to screen and provide brief interventions to patients in only a few minutes. This method helps not only to identify those patients who smoke, but also whether or not they are willing to make an attempt to quit.

Patients who are not ready to proceed with tobacco cessation may lack information regarding the hazards of tobacco use or the benefits of quitting, or have been discouraged by previous unsuccessful attempts.[19] Motivational interviewing can be used with these patients to encourage patients to consider cessation. Motivational interviewing focuses on the 5 Rs: relevance, risks, rewards, roadblocks, and repetition (**Fig. 2**). This patient-centered technique encourages self-identification of reasons for quitting, as well as to recognize personal factors that may help or hinder success.

Most patients will benefit from a combination of pharmacologic and nonpharmacologic (counseling) therapies.[19] Brief interventions, motivational interviewing, and careful review of past medical history and current medications will need to be considered when discussing the plan of care with the patient. Regular follow up can also help to ensure the patient will succeed.

PHARMACOLOGIC TREATMENTS
Nicotine Replacement Therapy

The US Food and Drug Administration has approved nicotine replacement therapy (NRT) as well as 2 non-nicotine medications, bupropion and varenicline, for first-line smoking cessation therapy.[19] Because nicotine is the primary substance responsible for withdrawal symptoms in patients attempting the quit smoking, NRT can be useful alone or in conjunction with other therapies. Common symptoms of nicotine withdrawal are listed in **Box 2**.[20] Nicotine withdrawal symptoms can begin within hours of the last cigarette and are at maximal intensity for the first week.[10] Most symptoms resolve over 3 to 4 weeks.

There are 5 forms of NRT available in the United States: a transdermal patch, chewing gum, lozenges, inhalers, and nasal spray preparations.[21] Inhalers and nasal sprays are only available by prescription; the patch, gum, and lozenges can be purchased over the counter. Nicotine dose and frequency of use varies by replacement route, which is summarized in **Table 2**. The average cigarette delivers 1 to 3 mg of nicotine; therefore, a pack per day smoker would absorb 20 to 60 mg of nicotine per day.[22] Most adverse effects related to NRT are related to local irritation to the mucosa or skin, but nausea and insomnia may also occur.[19] Insomnia is most likely to occur with the patch; if so, the patient can remove the patch at bedtime and replace in upon waking.

All forms of NRT allow for nicotine to enter the bloodstream, absorbed either through the oral or nasal mucosa or transdermally as with the patch.[21] From the bloodstream, the nicotine stimulates the nicotinic receptors in the ventral tegmental area of the brain, resulting in the release of dopamine in the nucleus acumbens.[23] Through

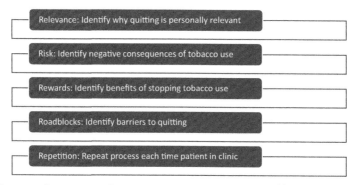

Relevance: Identify why quitting is personally relevant

Risk: Identify negative consequences of tobacco use

Rewards: Identify benefits of stopping tobacco use

Roadblocks: Identify barriers to quitting

Repetition: Repeat process each time patient in clinic

Fig. 2. The 5 Rs of motivational interviewing. (*Adapted from* Ref.[19])

Box 2
Symptoms of nicotine withdrawal (DSM-V)

- Irritability, frustration, or anger
- Anxiety
- Difficulty concentrating
- Increased appetite
- Restlessness
- Depressed mood
- Insomnia

Data from Ref.[20]

---

mucosal absorption, nicotine will reach the receptors in the brain within minutes. Nicotine patches allow for slow and controlled dosing of nicotine, which is helpful in decreasing cravings and withdrawal symptoms, but does not address any of the behavioral aspects of smoking. Combining the patch with a lower dose immediate release form of NRT, such as 2-mg nicotine gum or lozenges, has been shown to improve results. The recommended duration of NRT varies slightly by formulation, but is generally between 2 and 6 months.[19] During that period of time, the patient should be encouraged to decrease their nicotine dosage. It should be noted that some successful quitters use NRT products beyond the recommended timeframe. Although continued nicotine addiction is possible, the use of these products is considered safter than continued tobacco use.[21]

Contraindications to NRT are few. In pregnancy and breastfeeding, all nicotine should be avoided.[23] However, the maternal risk and risk to fetus and infant are great from tobacco use, so in pregnant or breastfeeding patients who are not able to quit without pharmacologic support, NRT has been recommend outside of the United States. However, the US Preventive Services Task Force has determined that there is insufficient evidence to calculate whether the benefits offset the harms of NRT or other pharmaceuticals for tobacco cessation during pregnancy.[24] Therefore, the recommendation is that when a pregnant patient is identified as a tobacco user as part of brief intervention, behavioral interventions for smoking cessation should be provided.

For patients under the age of 18 to access NRT, a prescription is required.[25] The American Academy of Pediatrics recommends considering off-label use of NRT in adolescents who are moderately or severely addicted to nicotine, because these products are not approved by the US Food and Drug Administration for use in youth. In limited research studies, there is no evidence of harm from NRT in patients less than 18 years of age.[26,27] Furthermore, NRT combined with behavioral support has been shown to be effective for tobacco cessation in adolescents.[28] Compliance with NRT in adolescents can be problematic[29]; the argument could be made that issues with NRT compliance is not unique to adolescents.

NRT is considered safe in patients with stable CVD.[23] In patients with unstable angina, acute myocardial infarction, and acute stroke, NRT should be used with caution because nicotine is a vasoconstrictor. Continued smoking poses a greater health risk than NRT to patients with stable CVD; preparations that are more easily reversable such as lozenges or gum should be used over patches. Non-nicotine medications will be discussed elsewhere in this article and are summarized in **Table 3**.

| Table 2 |||
| NRT formulations available in the United States |||
Route	How Supplied	Typical Use
Patch	7 mg, 14 mg, 21 mg	Patch replaced every 24 h
Gum	2 mg, 4 mg	Start with 1 piece of gum every 1–2 h
Lozenge	2 mg, 4 mg	Start with 1 lozenge every 1–2 h, do not exceed 20/d
Inhaler	10 mg/cartridge	6–16 cartridges per day
Nasal spray	0.5 mg/actuation	1 spray each nostril, 10–12 times per day

Data from Refs.[19–22]

Bupropion

Bupropion is a prescription medication used for smoking cessation originally marketed as an antidepressant.[22] The exact mechanism of action is unknown, but bupropion is thought to be mediated by noradrenergic and/or dopaminergic mechanisms, which may help to alleviate some symptoms of withdrawal. Medication is initiated at 150 mg/d, and increased to twice daily after 3 days; the maximum recommend dose of bupropion is 300 mg/d.[30] Bupropion is often initiated 1 to 2 weeks before quitting smoking, and is generally prescribed for 7 to 12 weeks, but maintenance dosing can be used for up to 6 months.[19,22] It can be combined with NRT to improve chances of patient success. The most common side effects include dry mouth and insomnia. There is a small risk of seizure with this medication, so it should not be prescribed to patients with a history of seizure. Upon termination of therapy, patients should be weaned off bupropion using a tapered dose over 1 to 2 weeks.

Varenicline

Varenicline is a partial agonist of the nicotinic receptor, inhibiting nicotine-induced dopamine release, decreasing reinforcement and psychological reward of smoking.[31] Patients are titrated up from 0.5 mg/d to 1.0 mg twice daily, at which point smoking cessation is initiated.[19] The duration of treatment is 3 to 6 months. Dosage should be decreased in patients with severe renal impairment or in those patients requiring dialysis. The most frequently reported adverse effect is nausea (9%–28%), but using a titration dosing schedule can help minimize this side effect.[32] Insomnia is also frequently reported (12%–21%), especially in the first 4 weeks of treatment, but becomes less common as treatment continues. Other common adverse effects include headache and abnormal dreams. There have been postmarketing reports of exacerbations of previously stable psychiatric disorders, and as such the US Food and Drug Administration has recommended screening for mood or behavior changes or worsening of preexisting psychiatric illness in patients currently taking varenicline and in those who have recently discontinued treatment.

Other Medications

There are 2 second-line therapies for tobacco cessation approved for use in the United States, namely, nortriptyline and clonidine, often used in combination with NRT.[19] These medications are generally used for patients unable to use first-line medications owing to contraindications or in patients where first-line treatment has been unsuccessful. Nortriptyline, a tricyclic antidepressant, has been shown to be effective for tobacco cessation in smokers with and without a history of depression, and success rates increase when combined with NRT.[22] The most commonly encountered adverse effects of nortriptyline include tachycardia, blurred vision, urinary retention,

Table 3
Oral medications for smoking cessation

Medication	Dosage/Duration	Common Adverse Effects	Contraindications
Bupropion	150 mg/d for 3 d, increase to 150 mg BID Start 1–2 wk before quit date Treat for 7–12 wk	Dry mouth, insomnia	Avoid in patients with history of seizure
Varenicline	Days 1–3: 0.5 mg/d Days 4–7: 0.5 mg BID Day 8 on: 1 mg BID Start 1 wk before quit date Treat for 12–24 wk	Nausea, insomnia, headache, abnormal dreams	Decrease dose in severe renal impairment, those requiring dialysis Screen for preexisting psychiatric diagnosis
Nortriptyline	25 mg/d, may titrate up to 75–100 mg/d Start 1–2 wk before quit date Continue for ≥12 wk after quit date	Tachycardia, blurred vision, urinary retention, dry mouth, constipation, orthostatic hypotension	Do not use with conditions or medications that prolong QT interval
Clonidine	0.1 mg/d, may increase to 0.15–0.75 mg/d if needed	Constipation, dizziness, drowsiness, dry mouth	Risk of rebound hypertension if discontinued suddenly

Abbreviation: BID, 2 times per day.
Data from Refs.[19,22,30–34]

dry mouth, constipation, and orthostatic hypotension.[33] Generally, the patient is started on 25 mg/d 1 to 2 weeks before the quit date and titrated up to 75 to 100 mg/d. Patient can be weaned from medication 12 weeks after quit date.

The alpha-adrenergic agonist clonidine has been shown to decrease symptoms of tobacco withdrawal.[22] Patients should be started at 0.1 mg/d, which can be increased to 0.15 to 0.75 mg/d if necessary, to control symptoms.[34] Common adverse effects of clonidine include constipation, dizziness, drowsiness, and dry mouth. Some patients may experience more severe effects of allergic reaction, bradycardia, and hypertension or hypotension, so clinicians should carefully screen patients before using clonidine for tobacco cessation treatment.[22]

NONPHARMACOLOGIC TREATMENTS

Behavioral interventions, alone or combined with pharmacologic treatments, can greatly increase the likelihood of successful tobacco use cessation.[24] Examples include, but are not limited to, in-person behavioral support, telephone counseling, and self-help materials. These interventions can be delivered in primary care or can occur in referred community settings. Cessation rates improve with even brief interventions, with studies showing that counseling for less than 3 minutes can be effective, although multiple sessions should be provided.[19] Group and individual counseling are effective and should include training in problem solving skills to help smokers recognize situations that increase their risk of smoking and to develop coping skills to overcome barriers to quitting.

Box 3
Online resources for tobacco cessation

www.cdc.gov/quit

www.fda.gov/tobacco-products/health-information/tobacco-public-health-resources

www.smokefree.gov

www.tobaccofreekids.org.

One easily accessible form of telephone counseling, which is often free to the caller, are tobacco quitlines.[35] The first tobacco quitline was developed by the US National Cancer Institute in the 1980s, and since residents of all 50 states, the District of Columbia, and the territories of Puerto Rico and Guam have access to tobacco quitlines, centrally available at 1-800-QUIT-NOW.[36,37] These services are also available in Spanish, Mandarin, Cantonese, Korean, and Vietnamese. Additionally, telephone quitlines may have companion websites and smart phone apps. Some states' quitlines can also help to provide the patient with tobacco cessation pharmacologic treatments. Print materials can easily be incorporated into counseling strategies and are widely available to clinicians so that they may provide self-help materials to their patients.[38] Websites that can be used as resources are listed in **Box 3**.

SUMMARY

Prevention and cessation strategies need to be multifaceted. Health care providers must consider many factors, including the patient's age, ethnicity, socioeconomic status, presence of comorbidities, and health care literacy level. Because tobacco use represents a modifiable risk factor for a multitude of diseases, screening for use and evaluating patients for appropriate cessation strategies, as well as advocating for tobacco prevention need to be on the forefront. The tobacco epidemic has long been sustained by tobacco industry. The general public has been misled deliberately regarding the risks of tobacco use. Advertising by tobacco companies has been shown to lead to adolescent and young adult experimentation and continued smoking behaviors.

CLINICS CARE POINTS

- Smoking is the leading cause of preventable death in the United States.
- Tobacco users are at risk for developing smoking-related cancers and smoking-related disease, and have increased risk for all-cause mortality.
- Nicotine dependence is the primary drive for continued smoking.
- Tobacco prevention efforts should be aimed at youth and young adults, because most smokers start using tobacco before the age of 18 years.
- Screening for tobacco use should be part of every patient encounter.
- Combining pharmacologic and nonpharmacologic treatments for tobacco cessation improves likelihood of success.

DISCLOSURE

The author has nothing to disclose.

REFERENCES

1. The health consequences of smoking— 50 years of progress: a report of the surgeon general. Atlanta: Department of Health and Human Services, Centers for Disease Control and Prevention, National Center for Chronic Disease Prevention and Health Promotion, Office on Smoking and Health; 2014.
2. Xu X, Bishop EE, Kennedy SM, et al. Annual healthcare spending attributable to cigarette smoking: an update. Am J Prev Med 2015;48(3):326–33.
3. Burden of cigarette use in the U.S; Current cigarette smoking among U.S. adults aged 18 years and older. 2020. Available at: https://www.cdc.gov/tobacco/campaign/tips/resources/data/cigarette-smoking-in-united-states.html. Accessed December 18, 2020.
4. Kasza KA, Ambrose BK, Conway KP, et al. Tobacco-Product Use by Adults and Youths in the United States in 2013 and 2014. N Engl J Med 2017;376(4):342–53.
5. Behavioral health trends in the United States: results from the 2014 national survey on drug use and health. 2015. Available at: http://www.samhsa.gov/data/. Accessed January 08, 2021.
6. Hu SS, Neff L, Agaku IT, et al. Tobacco product use among adults—United States, 2013-2014. MMWR Morb Mortal Wkly Rep 2016;65(27):685–91.
7. Wang TW, Asman K, Gentzke AS, et al. Tobacco product use among adults— United States, 2017. MMWR Morb Mortal Wkly Rep 2018;67(44):1225–32.
8. Kalkhoran S, Benowitz NL, Rigotti NA. Reprint of: prevention and treatment of tobacco use; JACC health promotion series. J Am Coll Cardiol 2018;72(23): 2964–79.
9. Smoking & Tobacco use; Economic Trends in tobacco. Available at: https://www.cdc.gov/tobacco/data_statistics/fact_sheets/economics/econ_facts/index.htm. Accessed December 18, 2020.
10. Jarvis MJ. ABC of smoking cessation; Why people smoke. BMJ 2004;328:277–9.
11. Smoking and Health. Report of the advisory Committee to the surgeon general of the public health service. Washington, DC: U.S. Department of Health Education and Welfare, Public Health Service; 1964.
12. Balough E, Patlak M, Nass SJ. Reducing tobacco-related cancer incidence & mortality; workshop summary. Washington DC: The National Academies Press; 2013.
13. Bonnie RJ, Kwan LY, Stratton KR, editors. Public health implications of raising the minimum age of legal access to tobacco products. Washington, DC: National Academies Press; 2015.
14. U.S. Department of Health Human Services. Preventing tobacco use among youth and young adults: a report of the surgeon general. Atlanta, GA: U.S. Department of Health and Human Ser- vices, Centers for Disease Control and Prevention, National Center for Chronic Disease Prevention and Health Promotion, Office on Smoking and Health; 2012. p. 3.
15. Wellman RJ, Sugarman DB, DiFranza JR, et al. The extent to which tobacco marketing and tobacco use in films contribute to children's use of tobacco: a meta-analysis. Arch Pediatr Adolesc Med 2006;160:1285–96.
16. Rose SW, Anesetti-Rothermel A, Elmasry H, et al. Young adult non-smokers' exposure to real-world tobacco marketing: results of an ecological momentary assessment pilot study. BMC Res Notes 2017;10:435.
17. Roberts ME, Keller-Hamilton B, Hinton A, et al. The magnitude and impact of tobacco marketing exposure in adolescents' day-to-day lives: an ecological momentary assessment (EMA) study. Addict Behav 2019;88:144–9.

18. Chaloupka FJ. Macro-social influences: the effects of prices and tobacco-control policies on the demand for tobacco products. Nicotine Tob Res 1999;1(Suppl 1): S105–9.
19. Fiore MC, Jaen CR, Baker TB, et al. A clinical practice guideline for treating tobacco use and dependance: 2008 update; A U.S. public health service report. Am J Prev Med 2008;35(2):158–76.
20. Substance-related and addictive disorders. In: Diagnostic and statistical manual of mental disorders: DSM-5. Arlington: American Psychiatric Association; 2013.
21. Stead LF, Perera R, Bullen C, et al. Nicotine replacement therapy for smoking cessation. Cochrane Database Syst Rev 2008;(1):CD000146.
22. Henningfield JE, Fant RV, Buchhalter AR, et al. Pharacotherapy for nicotine dependance. CA Cancer J Clin 2005;55:281–99.
23. Molyneux A. ABC of smoking cessation: nicotine replacement therapy. BMJ 2004; 328:454–6.
24. U.S. Preventative Services Task Force. Behavioral and pharmacotherapy interventions for tobacco smoking cessation in adults, including pregnant women: recommendation statement. Am Fam Physician 2016;93(10):860A-860G.
25. Supporting youth who are addicted to nicotine: advice for pediatricians. Available at: https://downloads.aap.org/RCE/Factsheet_Supporting_Youth_Addicted_to_Nicotine.pdf. Accessed January 08, 2021.
26. US Preventive Services Task Force. Final recommendation statement: tobacco use in children and adolescents: primary care interventions 2013. Available at: https://www.uspreventiveservicestaskforce.org/Page/Document/RecommendationStatementFinal/tobacco-use-in-children-and-adolescents-primary-care-interventions. Accessed January 08, 2021.
27. US Preventive Services Task Force. Draft recommendation statement: prevention and cessation of tobacco use in children and adolescents: primary care interventions 2020. Available at: https://www.uspreventiveservicestaskforce.org/uspstf/recommendation/tobacco-and-nicotine-use-prevention-in-children-and-adolescents-primary-care-interventions. Accessed January 08, 2021.
28. Swanson AN, Shoptaw S, Heinzerling KG, et al. Up in smoke? A preliminary open-label trial of nicotine replacement therapy and cognitive behavioral motivational enhancement for smoking cessation among youth in Los Angeles. Subst Use Misuse 2013;48:1553–62.
29. Scherphof CS, van den Eijnden RJJM, Lugtig P, et al. Adolescents' use of nicotine replacement therapy for smoking cessation: predictors of compliance trajectories. Psychopharmacology 2014;231:1743–52.
30. UpToDate. Bupropion: drug information. Available at: https://www.uptodate.com/contents/bupropion-drug-information?search=bupropion&source=panel_search_result&selectedTitle=1~145&usage_type=panel&kp_tab=drug_general&display_rank=1. Accessed January 08, 2021.
31. Rollema H, Chambers LK, Coe JW, et al. Pharmacological profile of the $\alpha 4\beta 2$ nicotinic acetylcholine receptor partial agonist varenicline, an effective smoking cessation aid. Neuropharmacology 2007;52:985–94.
32. Daubney Garrison G, Dugan SE. Varnicline: a first-line treatment option for smoking cessation. Clin Ther 2009;31(3):463–91.
33. UpToDate. Nortriptyline: drug information. Available at: https://www.uptodate.com/contents/nortriptyline-drug-information?search=nortriptyline&source=panel_search_result&selectedTitle=1~98&usage_type=panel&kp_tab=drug_general&display_rank=1#F202717. Accessed January 08, 2021.

34. Medscape. Clonidine. Available at: https://reference.medscape.com/drug/catapres-tts-clonidine-342382. Accessed January 08, 2021.

35. All quitline facts. 2009. Available at: https://cdn.ymaws.com/www.naquitline.org/resource/resmgr/ql_about_facts/2008_quitline_facts_qa_final.pdf.   Accessed January 08, 2021.

36. Anderson CM, Zhu S. Tobacco quitlines: looking back and looking ahead. Tob Control 2007;16(Suppl 1):i81–6.

37. Five reasons why calling a quitline can be key to your success. Available at: https://www.cdc.gov/tobacco/campaign/tips/quit-smoking/quitline/index.html. Accessed January 08, 2021.

38. Patnode CP, Henderson JT, Thompson JH, et al. Behavioral counseling and pharmacotherapy interventions for tobacco cessation in adults, including pregnant women: a review of reviews for the U.S. Preventive Services Task Force. Ann Intern Med 2015;163(8):608–21.

Nutrition Food Policy Guidelines

What Should Patients Eat?

Joel G. McReynolds, PA-C, MPAS, CAQ-Orthopedic Surgery[a,*],
Nguyen H. Park, MS, PA-C, DFAAPA[b], Matthew Wright, MS, PA-C, RD[c]

KEYWORDS

- Nutrition • Guidelines • Nutrigenomics • Epidemiology • Prevention
- Chronic disease

KEY POINTS

- Public health policy should be personalized for each patient's medical history
- The use of optimal nutrition, with appropriate caloric intake, can often treat and prevent chronic disease
- Nutrient-dense foods are preferred.
- Highly processed foods and sugar-sweetened beverages should be avoided.

INTRODUCTION

Throughout history, public health nutrition has served to shape nutrition food policy, beginning primarily as a population-level approach to disease prevention, health promotion, and addressing malnutrition and undernutrition.[1] For example, in the early 1800s, public health policies formed public school lunch programs, milk stations, and state and local health departments. Primarily in the United States, the focus began with addressing infant and child morbidity and mortality, and diseases caused by nutritional deficiencies such as rickets and scurvy. As industrialization increased, nutrition food policy has shifted toward disease prevention from dietary excesses with the increased availability of nutrient-poor foods and the resultant obesity epidemic, which has been implicated in diet-related noncommunicable diseases such as diabetes, atherosclerotic cardiovascular disease, hypertension, and certain types of cancers.

[a] New West Sports Medicine and Orthopedic Surgery, 2810 West 35th Street, Kearney, NE 68845, USA; [b] 413 River Bend Road, Great Falls, VA 22066, USA; [c] Rutgers University School of Health Professions, Physician Assistant Program, 675 Hoes Lane West, 6th Floor, Piscataway, NJ 08854, USA
* Corresponding author.
E-mail address: joelgmcreynolds@gmail.com

Physician Assist Clin 7 (2022) 181–190
https://doi.org/10.1016/j.cpha.2021.08.008
2405-7991/22/© 2021 Elsevier Inc. All rights reserved.
physicianassistant.theclinics.com

Nutrition food policy is a global concern, often addressing food shortages with war and famine in less developed nations and shifting as noted elsewhere in this article, to focus on chronic diseases caused by decreased physical activity and poor dietary intake in developing countries and countries in transition as they become more industrialized and urban. International organizations such as the World Health Organization, World Public Health Nutrition Association, and the Food First Information and Action Network International, review nutrition food policy from a public health perspective taking into account the global food economy. Most recently, in December of 2020, the World Health Organization pronounced 2021 to 2030 to be the Decade of Healthy Aging, adding the health concerns of a rapidly aging population to their focus in public health research.[2]

In the United States, the Food and Drug Administration, which was established in 1906, and its Center for Food Safety and Applied Nutrition, the Department of Agriculture, established in 1862, and its extramural science-funding agency, the National Institute of Food and Agriculture, and the Centers for Disease Control and Prevention play a role in establishing nutrition food policy, ensuring food safety, and supporting evidence-based nutrition epidemiology research.

As data from more epidemiologic studies such as the Centers for Disease Control and Prevention's National Center for Health Statistics' National Health and Nutrition Examination Survey,[3] the Framingham Heart Study,[4] and the Jackson Heart Study,[5] are collected and analyzed, the focus has shifted to improving measurable outcomes based on evidence-based studies, and recommendations from medical societies or associations for treating specific populations of patients emerged. Included in this article are guidelines from numerous medical associations based on studies like these to help physician assistants to provide guidance to patients, in the prevention and treatment of chronic diseases, in recovery from surgical procedures (Enhanced Recovery After Surgery), and in the promotion of healthy aging.

DIETARY GUIDELINES FOR AMERICANS

The Dietary Guidelines for Americans (DGA)[6] are established by a committee of recognized nutrition experts sponsored by the US Department of Agriculture and the Department of Health and Human Services. Guidelines are updated in 5-year intervals with the specific objective of reviewing the most recent nutrition-related publications for health promotion and disease prevention. Completing the DGA[1] involves a systematic review process to identify and evaluate high-quality evidence supportive of beneficial nutrition practices across the lifespan.

The latest edition has continued the public and preventative health focus of the publication, as well as the emphasis on nutrient dense dietary patterns opposed to individual nutrients.[7] DGAs are not intended to represent clinical practice guidelines to treat chronic, nutrition-related disease and instead provide a beneficial strategy for prevention. Similar to the previous publication, the 2020 to 2025 edition has delivered recommendations for distinct phases of life, including pregnancy and lactation, birth to 24 months, childhood and adolescence, adulthood, and older adulthood.[6] Threaded through each distinct stage of life, the DGA have established 4 primary goals in attempts to maximize health. For each period of the lifespan, individuals should attempt to follow a healthy eating pattern, customize nutrient-dense food and beverage choices reflective of culture and personal preferences, consume nutrient-dense foods while staying within calorie needs, and limit saturated fats, added sugars, sodium, and alcohol intake.[6,7]

Throughout the guidelines and in each individual phase of the lifespan the phrases "nutrient-dense" and "dietary pattern" are used in a specific fashion to promote maximum benefit in food and beverages consumed. The scientific panel has defined nutrient-dense foods as those foods that provide high-quality vitamins, minerals, and other healthful components while containing little added sugar, saturated fat, and sodium. "Dietary pattern" is representative of consistency in consuming nutrient-dense foods in proper amounts from all food groups.[6] Recommendations are subsequently delivered based on lifespan appropriate, nutrient-dense food choices.

NUTRITION FOR INFANTS AND TODDLERS

The infancy and toddler period is described as zero to 24 months of age.[7] With specific regard to the first 6 months of life, the consensus of the DGA scientific committee to maximize a baseline healthy dietary pattern is to exclusively provide human milk when possible.[6] Nutrient needs can largely be met with breastfeeding, with the exception of vitamin D.[6,7] Support for breastfeeding can be encouraged with the use of human donor milk as well as a breast pump when available, while concurrently providing 400 international units of vitamin D daily.[6] Breastfeeding, as determined by the scientific committee, has been associated with decreased rates of childhood atopy and obesity from age 2 and beyond; limited to moderate evidence exists demonstrating reduced risks of type 1 and 2 diabetes as well as cardiovascular disease when compared with no history of breastfeeding.[7]

Complementary nutrient-dense foods should be incorporated into a child's diet around 4 to 6 months of age. An emphasis should be placed on a wide variety of developmentally appropriate foods from all groups, including those rich in iron, to maximize nutrient delivery. Additionally, potentially allergenic foods should not be delayed in the first year of life. In particular, infants at high risk of peanut allergy should have peanuts introduced into their diet within 4 to 6 months to decrease the likelihood of developing a peanut allergy.[6,7] However, parents and caregivers should be discouraged from providing cow's milk or fortified soy as a milk replacement before 12 months of age, although yogurt and cheeses are considered developmentally acceptable foods. Other foods recommended to avoid in the first year of life are those with a high sodium content, including many processed meats and salty snacks, as well as added sugars, including fruit juice and other sugar-sweetened beverages. One hundred percent fruit juice may be introduced after 12 months of age, although benefits obtained from whole fruits outweigh juice consumption.[6]

Beyond the first year of life, nutrient needs should be met with a healthy dietary pattern. Although formula is not generally recommended beyond 12 months of age, children tend to drink less human milk in their second year as well.[6] A wide variety of nutrient-dense foods are essential to meet needs in the second year of life. An emphasis should be placed on whole fruits, vegetables, whole grains, lean meats, dairy, and oils. If seafood is consumed as a lean protein source, fish including lower mercury levels as defined by the Food and Drug Administration are encouraged.[8]

CHILDHOOD, ADOLESCENTS, AND ADULTS

The DGAs[6] recommend similar dietary patterns for children and adults, extending healthful routines established in the infancy and toddler ages.[6] Although calorie and nutrient requirements vary widely by age and sex in these lifespans, prevention of chronic nutrition-related disease is maximized by focusing on nutrient-dense foods consumed on a consistent basis. However, according to Healthy Eating Index[9] scores used in the DGAs,[1] the vast majority of American children and adolescents exceed recommended intakes of added sugars, saturated fat, and sodium with increasing intakes from childhood to adolescence.[6] Similar patterns are seen in adults, with the majority not meeting goals of the dietary guidelines. A strong understanding of the general dietary habits of each phase of the lifespan allows for unique opportunities and methods for clinicians to provide support for nutrient-dense dietary patterns.

Clinicians should be attentive to the amount of sugar-sweetened beverages their child and adolescent patients are consuming, including fruit juices. Children and adolescents, more so than other age groups, consume these food products more frequently than recommended. Additionally, concern exists for the inadequate intake of vitamin D, calcium, and dietary fiber.[6,7] Children and parents should be counseled to decrease the frequency with which sugar-sweetened beverages are consumed and to meet age-specific recommendations for vegetables, fruit, whole grain, and low-fat dairy intake (**Table 1**).[6] Dietary patterns for these age groups tend to reflect the home eating environment. Clinicians recommending dietary adjustments for their young child and adolescent populations should therefore encourage healthy adjustments be made across all family members in the household.[6]

Special considerations for adult and older adults are similar to those for children. Of particular concern continues to be low fiber, calcium, and vitamin D intake as well as high consumption of sodium, saturated fat, and added sugars.[6,7] Clinicians focusing on dietary adjustments to increase nutrient-dense foods can encourage adults to meet recommended vegetable, fruit and grain intake (see **Table 1**) to meet daily fiber needs. Specifically focusing on fresh vegetables and fruits as well as whole grains as opposed to processed and ready-prepared foods aids in decreasing sources of dietary sodium and added sugars. Recommendations to decrease saturated fat and ensure adequate calcium and vitamin D include focusing on lean, lower fat sources of protein and dairy foods, such as fortified skim or soy milk as opposed to whole or 2% milk, and very lean ground beef opposed to 80% lean.[6,7]

There is particular concern for older adults to meet protein recommendations secondary to age-related sarcopenia. Clinicians should pay particular attention to dietary intakes of protein for their patients who are 60 years of age or older, particularly if they have experienced unexplained weight loss. Concurrently, ability to absorb vitamin B_{12} may decrease with aging which can be mitigated by the addition of food sources high in vitamin B_{12}, such as animal proteins, and fortified foods, such as breakfast cereals.[6]

Alcohol has not been included in the DGA recommendations, although it is recognized, given the frequency of consumption by American adults. For adults who do not consume alcohol, particularly older adults, it is not recommended to begin at this life stage given the added risks of falls and motor vehicle accidents.[6,7] For adults who do consume alcohol, clinicians should strongly encourage no more than moderate intake (2 drinks per day for men, 1 drink per day for women).[6]

PREGNANCY AND LACTATION

Women who are pregnant or breastfeeding should follow a similar dietary pattern, incorporating nutrient-dense food selections as in other phases of the lifespan. Calories increase above baseline requirements in pregnancy and during breastfeeding, which can be met with nutrient-dense food selections.[6] Critically important nutrients for fetal development include folic acid, iron, iodine, and choline. Folate requirements are increased to prevent neural tube defects in the developing fetus and clinicians should recommend that women of childbearing age, and those considering becoming pregnant, to begin a 400 to 800 μg daily supplement.[6,7] Iron needs increase in pregnancy as well, which can be met with consumption of heme and nonheme iron sources. Nonheme iron absorption, generally obtained from plant foods, can be enhanced with the concurrent consumption of vitamin C.[6] Iodine and choline are important for

Table 1
Recommended intakes across the lifespan

Age Range	Daily Vegetables, Cups/d	Daily Fruit, Cups/d	Daily Grains,[a] Ounces/d	Total Dairy, C/d	Total Protein, Ounces/d d
0–6 mo[b]	N/A	N/A	N/A	N/A	N/A
6–12 mo (4–6 mo to 1 y)	Introduce	Introduce	Introduce	Introduce	Introduce
12–23 mo	0.5–1.0	0.5–1.0	1.75–3.0	1.75–2.0	2.0
2–4 y	1.0–2.0	1.0–1.5	3.0–5.0	2.0–2.5	2.0–5.0
5–8 y	1.5–2.5	1.0–2.0	4.0–6.0	2.5	3.0–5.5
9–13 y	2.0–3.5 (M), 1.3–3.0 (F)	1.5–2.0 (M and F)	5.0–9.0 (M), 5.0–7.0 (F)	3.0 (M&F)	5.0–6.5 (M), 4.0–6.0 (F)
14–18 y	2.5–4.0 (M), 2.5–3.0 (F)	2.0–2.5 (M), 1.5–2.0 (F)	6.0–10.0 (M), 6.0–8.0 (F)	3.0 (M&F)	5.5–7.0 (M), 5.0–6.5 (F)
19–30 y	3.0–4.0 (M), 2.5–3.0 (F)	2.0–2.5 (M), 1.5–2.0 (F)	8.0–10.0 (M), 6.0–8.0 (F)	3.0 (M&F)	6.5–7.0 (M), 5.0–6.5 (F)
31–59 y	3.0–4.0 (M), 2.0–3.0 (F)	2.0–2.5 (M), 1.5–2.0 (F)	7.0–10.0 (M), 5.0–7.0 (F)	3.0 (M&F)	6.0–7.0 (M), 5.0–6.0 (F)
60 y and older	2.5–3.5 (M), 2.0–3.0 (F)	2.0 (M), 1.5–2.0 (F)	6.0–9.0 (M), 5.0–7.0 (F)	3.0 (M&F)	5.5–6.5 (M), 5.0–6.0 (F)
Pregnancy and lactation	2.5–3.5 (P&L)	1.5–2.5 (P&L)	6.0–10.0 (P&L)	3.0 (P&L)	5.0–7.0 (P&L)

Abbreviations: F, female; L, lactating; M, male; P, pregnancy.

[a] Emphasize whole grains.

[b] 0 to 6 mo of age (4–6 months) encouraged to meet all nutritional needs from human milk or formula.

neurocognitive and brain development during pregnancy. Clinicians can recommend regular intake of eggs, seafood from appropriate sources and amounts, and meats, as well as iodized salts when using table salt to help meet these requirements.[6,7]

NUTRITION AND CANCER PREVENTION

Nutrition guidelines from the American Cancer Society (ACS) have been published for the prevention of cancer.[10] Other agencies including the National Cancer Institute[11] and the American Institute for Cancer Research[3] have contributed additional information on specific cancer-related nutrition topics as well. The most recent practice guidelines from the ACS were published in 2020 and reflect current nutritional, epidemiologic, and randomized controlled trial data. The ACS's latest position statement[10] is strongly reflective of fundamental principles clinicians should use to educate their patients in cancer prevention and care.

DIET PATTERNS AND FOOD GROUPS

Nutrition and nutrition-related factors play an important role in the prevention of cancer. Recent evidence has demonstrated that 18.2% of cancer cases are associated with a combination of body weight, diet, alcohol consumption, and physical inactivity.[12] Healthy diet and exercise represent important methods to mitigate cancer development partially through the prevention of obesity and being overweight. This pattern is evident for a wide variety of cancers.[10]

A healthy dietary pattern should be emphasized to promote a normal body weight and decrease the risks of cancer. Patterns encouraged by the ACS[1] are similar to those described in the DGA's 2020 to 2025 edition,[6] and should more so be the focus of patient counseling than individual nutrients. Foods to encourage are those that are high in nutrients and aid in the maintenance of a healthy body weight. Emphasized highly by the ACS guidelines to be consumed are a variety of colorful fruits and vegetables, as well as whole grains. Decreases in red meat and processed meats, along with highly processed foods, sugar-sweetened beverages, and alcohol, should also be encouraged.[6] Of particular note, dietary patterns that are rich in plant foods and lower in processed foods have been associated with lower rates of both breast and colorectal cancers.[12] Similar recommendations have been made with regard to decreasing the consumption of processed and cured meats by the National Cancer Institute.[13]

Other dietary patterns demonstrating associations with a lower likelihood of cancer development (with the added bonus of preventing the number one chronic illness, cardiovascular disease) are the Mediterranean and DASH diet (Dietary Approaches to Stop Hypertension)[10] (**Table 2**). Both dietary patterns, as well as the DGAs,[6] emphasize greater consumption of nutrient-dense foods such as vegetables, fruits, and whole grain, while decreasing consumption of foods higher in sugar and saturated fats, aligning them well with the ACS recommendations. Other dietary strategies are explored in **Table 3**. Consistent evidence has demonstrates these patterns to be associated with reduced incidence of cancer, as well as all-cause mortality.[10]

Fruits, vegetables, and whole grains are all individually associated with lower rates of cancer.[10] Fruits and vegetables contain a variety of active compounds including vitamins, minerals, phytochemicals, flavonoids, and fiber that all likely contribute to decreased associations with a variety of cancers. Specifically, a lower incidence of breast and gastrointestinal cancers are noted with a higher intake of fruit and vegetables.[13,14] Additionally, whole grain consumption of at least 30 g/d is negatively associated with colorectal cancer rates.[10] Higher consumption of fruits, vegetables, and

Table 2
A Clinician's guide to healthy eating for cardiovascular disease prevention[17]

	DASH Diet	USDA Healthy Mediterranean	USDA Healthy Vegetarian Diet
Grains	6–8 servings daily	6 ounces daily, 2 whole and 2 refined	6 ounces daily, 3 whole and 3 refined
Vegetables	4–5 servings daily	2.5 cups daily	2.5 cups daily
Fruits	4–5 servings daily	2 cups daily	1.5 cups daily
Nuts, seeds, legumes	4–5 servings daily	1.0–2.0	4.0–6.0
Low-fat dairy	2–3 servings daily	6 ounces daily	3 ounces daily
Lean meats, poultry, fish	<6 ounces daily	2 ounces daily	2 ounces daily
Fats, oils	2–3 servings daily	24 g daily	24 g daily
Sweets, sugars	<5 servings weekly	Limit, no quantity specified	Limit, no quantity specified
Sodium	<2.3 g sodium daily	Limit, no quantity specified	Limit, no quantity specified
Alcohol	1 or less drink for women, 2 or less for men	Limit, no quantity specified	Limit, no quantity specified

Abbreviations: DASH, dietary approaches to stop hypertension; USDA, US Department of Agriculture.

whole grains also aid in achieving a nutrient-dense and calorie-appropriate dietary pattern, helping to prevent inappropriate weight gain and further decreasing the likelihood of cancer development.[6,10]

Added sugars and heavily processed foods are recommended to be limited or avoided in a cancer-protective dietary pattern. Although evidence from the ACS's[10] guidelines has noted that high glycemic foods are likely associated with higher endometrial cancer rates, sugar-sweetened foods frequently contribute to obesity and have an indirect association with all cancers. Similar trends in higher body weight and cancer risks are noted with heavily processed foods.[10]

Alcohol should also be of limited consumption or avoided altogether to decrease cancer risks. Alcohol has been considered the third major modifiable risk factor for cancer development after tobacco and obesity.[12] In evidence reviewed by the ACS, alcohol was found to be strongly associated with development of oropharyngeal, laryngeal, esophageal, liver, and colorectal cancers. It is recommended that if alcohol is consumed is should be in moderation based on sex (1 standard drink per day for women, 2 standard drinks per day for men.)[10,12]

DIABETES MELLITUS AND KIDNEY DISEASE GUIDELINES

As one of the most prevalent diet-related noncommunicable diseases, type 2 diabetes mellitus, and its host of other complications including chronic kidney disease, are widely seen in most physician assistant practices, no matter what field of medicine in which they practice. The Kidney Disease: Improving Global Outcomes (KDIGO) Clinical Practice Guideline for Diabetes Management in Chronic Kidney Disease[15] published in 2020 represents the first KDIGO guideline in this population. Patients with

Table 3
Dietary interventions and ACS[1] recommendations

Dietary Intervention	ACS Recommendation
Antioxidants, supplemental (vitamins C, E, carotenoids, etc)	No current recommendation[a]
Genetically modified crops	No current evidence indicating protective effect of increased risks
Gluten-free diet	No current evidence linked to reduced cancer rates[b]
Vegetarian/vegan diet	Associated with less cancer risk than typical Western diet[c]
Glycemic index/glycemic load	Diet patterns with frequent consumption of high glycemic carbohydrates associated with endometrial cancer
Juicing/cleansing and detox interventions	No evidence to support reduction in cancer risk
Organic foods	Little evidence to state reduced cancer risks. Early evidence for reduced non-Hodgkin lymphoma risk[d]
Non-nutritive sweeteners	No clear evidence to indicate an increased cancer risk

[a] Encourage to obtain through nutrient-dense dietary pattern.
[b] Whole grains containing gluten are associated with a lower risk of colorectal cancer; recommendation not made for those with celiac disease.
[c] Lower cancer risks compared with individuals who consume smaller amounts of animal protein is unknown.
[d] Results need to be replicated in additional trials.

type 2 diabetes mellitus and chronic kidney disease require a foundation of lifestyle interventions in addition to maximization of therapeutic options to decrease risk factors to progression to developing ASCAD and progression of chronic kidney disease.

Optimizing a patient's nutritional status can have major effects on glycemic control and, thereby, on disease progression. Major nutrition recommendations that physician assistants can incorporate into their care of patients with type 2 diabetes mellitus include an emphasis on an individualized diet high in vegetables, fruits, whole grains, fiber, legumes, plant-based proteins, unsaturated fats, and nuts, and lower in processed meats, refined carbohydrates, and sweetened beverages. The suggested protein intake is 0.8 g protein/kg (weight) per day for patients with diabetes type 2 and chronic kidney disease not treated with dialysis. Sodium intake of less than 2 g or less than 90 mmol daily or less than 5 g of sodium chloride daily are also recommended.

SUMMARY

An understanding of public health nutrition and food policy as well as how epidemiologic studies influence how these policies are formed, are key to understanding the backdrop of how nutrition recommendations have served and continue to serve to improve public health, and thus how this process can be translated into better health for individual patients. In looking toward the future of public health nutrition, nutrigenomics,[16] a field that encompasses nutritional genomics research into how diet and the genome may influence health, will likely play an increasingly important role in medicine. As this practice gains momentum, more individualized recommendations for nutrition based on personalized medicine will likely arise from the findings of studies such as the All of Us Research program and the genomic testing branches of the Framingham Heart Study and the Jackson Heart Study. In the interim, physician assistants can continue to rely on guidelines that are increasingly including more nutrition recommendations to provide quality care for their patients.

CLINICS CARE POINTS

- Public health nutrition policy is shaped by nutritional epidemiologic studies, which inform medical society and association guidelines.
- Nutrition guidelines based on public health nutrition policy can help to improve outcomes, decrease disease burden, and prevent morbidity and mortality.
- Physician assistants should use guidelines tailored to specific patient populations for nutrition recommendations, which can improve health outcomes.
- Caloric intake should be tailored on an individual basis.
- Nutrient-dense foods are preferred over processed and sugar-sweetened foods and beverages.
- Protein is essential to prevent sarcopenia.
- Nutrition is vital to prevent and treat chronic disease

DISCLOSURE

No commercial or financial conflicts of interest.

REFERENCES

1. Ridgway E, Baker P, Woods J, et al. Historical developments and paradigm shifts in public health nutrition science, guidance and policy actions: a narrative review. Nutrients 2019;11(3):531.
2. Decade of healthy ageing: baseline report. Geneva: World Health Organization; 2020.
3. Ahluwalia N, Dwyer J, Terry A, et al. Update on NHANES dietary data: focus on collection, release, analytical considerations, and uses to inform public policy. Adv Nutr 2016;7(1):121–34.
4. Andersson C, Johnson AD, Benjamin EJ, et al. 70-year legacy of the Framingham Heart Study. Nat Rev Cardiol 2019;16(11):687–98.
5. Gao Y, Hickson DA, Talegawkar S, et al. Influence of individual life course and neighbourhood socioeconomic position on dietary intake in African Americans: the Jackson Heart Study. BMJ Open 2019;9(3):e025237.
6. U.S. Department of Agriculture and U.S. Department of Health and Human Services. Dietary guidelines for Americans, 2020-2025. 9th edition 2020. Available at: DietaryGuidelines.gov. Accessed January 11, 2021.
7. Dietary Guidelines Advisory Committee. Scientific report of the 2020 dietary guidelines advisory committee: advisory report to the secretary of agriculture and the secretary of health and human Services. Washington, DC: U.S. Department of Agriculture, Agricultural Research Service; 2020.
8. Advice about eating fish. FDA.gov. Available at: https://www.fda.gov/food/consumers/advice-about-eating-fish. Accessed January 11, 2021.

9. Healthy eating Index scores for Americans. FNS.USDA.gov. Available at: https://www.fns.usda.gov/hei-scores-americans. Accessed January 18, 2021.

10. Rock CL, Thomson C, Gansler T, et al. American Cancer Society guideline for diet and physical activity for cancer prevention. CA Cancer J Clin 2020;70(4):245–71.

11. National Cancer Institute. Red meat and processed meat consumption. 2021. Available at: https://progressreport.cancer.gov/prevention/red_meat. Accessed January 11, 2021.

12. Islami F, Goding Sauer A, Miller KD, et al. Proportion and number of cancer cases and deaths attributable to potentially modifiable risk factors in the United States. CA Cancer J Clin 2018;68:31–54.

13. World Cancer Research Fund & American Institute for Cancer Research. Whole grains, vegetables and fruit and the risk of cancer 2021. Available at: https://www.wcrf.org/dietandcancer/exposures/wholegrains-veg-fruit.

14. Bakker MF, Peeters PH, Klaasen VM, et al. Plasma carotenoids, vitamin C, tocopherols, and retinol and the risk of breast cancer in the European Prospective Investigation into cancer and nutrition cohort. Am J Clin Nutr 2016;103:454–64.

15. de Boer IH, Caramori ML, Chan JCN, et al. Executive summary of the 2020 KDIGO diabetes management in CKD guideline: evidence-based advances in monitoring and treatment. Kidney Int 2020;98(4):839–48.

16. Di Renzo L, Gualtieri P, Romano L, et al. Role of personalized nutrition in chronic-degenerative diseases. Nutrients 2019;11(8):1707.

17. Pallazola VA, Davis DM, Whelton SP, et al. A clinician's guide to healthy eating for cardiovascular disease prevention. Mayo Clin Proc Inn Qual Outcomes 2019;3:251–67.

COVID-19

Salt in the Wound of Health Care Inequality and the Cause of a New Health Care Disparity

Sarah Pieper, MPAS, PA-C

KEYWORDS

- COVID-19 • Health care disparity • Health inequality
- Nosocomial COVID-19 infections • Non–COVID-19 health conditions

INTRODUCTION

Being an emergency room (ER) PA in a rural community, I, unfortunately, see firsthand the sad stories, the impact, and the faces of health care disparity. However, like almost every other American, the year 2020 would be like no other for my family. My mother would face job loss and a new status, low socioeconomic status. She would become part of a statistical, an American of low socioeconomic status to contract COVID-19. She would also lose her health care coverage, diminishing her access to health care. All of this could be traced back to the indirect pain COVID-19 would inflict on the economy of my small hardworking hometown, forcing the local paper mill to close. If this was happening to my family, what was happening to those already fighting an uphill battle of health care despair before the pandemic?

Not only would my family face job loss and the issues thereof, my aunt would also be diagnosed with stage IV melanoma. Her diagnosis, and ultimately her time-sensitive treatment, would be delayed by 2 months because of the direct burden of the pandemic on the health care delivery system and on nonemergent procedures. Was COVID-19 opening up a new health care disparity wound? What was happening to those with chronic, time-sensitive medical conditions and those who rely on regular medical treatments? What effects would COVID-19-related barriers and delays in receiving adequate and timely care for non–COVID-19-related medical needs have on these patients? Not to mention, what effect would the pandemic have on routine medical screening examinations and routine screening procedures? How was COVID-19 going to affect medical conditions that are found during routine screenings if we were not screening patients? How would patient hesitancy to receive medical care due to the risks of contracting COVID-19 have on overall outcomes and mortality for non–COVID-19-related medical conditions?

Concordia University Wisconsin, 12800 N Lake Shore Drive, Mequon, WI 53097, USA
E-mail address: Haraslp3@gmail.com

Physician Assist Clin 7 (2022) 191–199
https://doi.org/10.1016/j.cpha.2021.08.009
2405-7991/22/© 2021 Elsevier Inc. All rights reserved.

physicianassistant.theclinics.com

COVID-19 AND RACE: SALT IN AN ALREADY OPEN WOUND OF HEALTH CARE DISPARITY

We know that COVID-19 did not create health care inequalities, but it has put salt in the open wound of health care inequality among racial groups in the United States. Just as the measles epidemic from 1989 to 1991, just like the yellow fever epidemic in 1792, COVID-19 would write a new page in public health with the same message. It would disproportionately impact those of color. As per the Centers for Disease Control (CDC) statistics[1] from November 2020, cases of COVID-19 would be 2.6 × higher in African Americans than in White, non-Hispanic persons. Hospitalizations would be 4.6 × higher and deaths would be 2.1 × higher among African Americans than among White non-Hispanic persons. The higher rates of cases, hospitalizations, and death from COVID-19 would also be higher among American Indian/Alaskan Natives and Hispanic/Latino persons. See **Fig. 1** and **Table 1** from CDC surveillance data. As of Nov 13, 2020, the most up-to-date CDC surveillance data for the rate of hospitalization are as follows: Demonstrating the disproportionate complications in the people of color[1]

- 465.4/100,000 for Hispanic or Latino
- 459.3/100,000 for American Indian or Alaskan Native
- 429.3/100,000 for non-Hispanic Black
- 114.6/100,000 for non-Hispanic White

In a retrospective cohort study reported in an article published in the *Journal of Racial and Ethnic Health Disparities*,[2] data demonstrate higher rates of hospitalization and mortality in racial minorities with COVID-19. This study looked at 734 hospitalized patients from 3/10/20 to 4/13/20 in their affiliated NYC hospitals. Data demonstrated that Blacks in Brooklyn were twice as likely to require hospitalization for COVID-19 (42.9/100,000) compared with White patients (22.7/100,000). Hispanics had an increased risk of inpatient mortality [hazard ratio (HR) = 1.84%; 95% confidence interval (CI) = 1.21–2.80; P = .005] along with Asian patients (HR = 2.06%; 95% CI = 1.08–3.93; P = .03). Blacks were also disproportionally a higher percentage of the COVID-19-related deaths than White patients.

DISCUSSION: WHAT CAN WE DO AS HEALTH CARE PROVIDERS
Key Points

- The reasons for racial disparity in COVID-19 hospitalization and mortality are multifactorial, thus so is the solution.

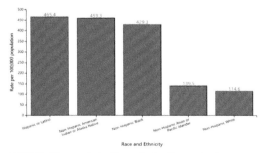

Fig. 1. Age-adjusted COVID-19-associated hospitalization rates by race and ethnicity-COVID-NET, March 1–November 14, 2020. (*From* https://www.cdc.gov/coronavirus/2019-ncov/covid-data/covidview/index.html.)

Table 1				
CDC death and hospitalization data by race				
Rate Ratios Compared to White, Non-Hispanic Persons	American Indian or Alaska Native, Non-Hispanic Persons	Asian, Non-Hispanic Persons	Black or African American, Non-Hispanic Persons	Hispanic or Latino Persons
Cases[1]	2.8 × higher	1.1 × higher	2.6 × higher	2.8 × higher
Hospitalization[2]	5.3 × higher	1.3 ×higher	4.7 × higher	4.6 × higher
Death[3]	1 4 × higher	No Increase	2.1 × higher	1.1 × higher

Race and ethnicity are risk markers for other underlying conditions that impact health – including socioeconomic status, access to health care, and increased exposure to the virus due to occupation (e.g., frontline, essential, and critical infrastructure workers).
From https://www.cdc.gov/coronavirus/2019-ncov/covid-data/investigations-discovery/hospitalization-death-by-race-ethnicity.html.

- People of color are at a higher risk of losing their job because of the economy related to the effect of COVID-19. There are state and federal grants to help displaced workers that we can provide information for.[3]
- It is known that people of color may not trust their medical provider or medical system. We need to increase our cultural understanding with institutional training engaging all medical professionals.[4]
- Encourage a safe environment that embraces cultural humility.
- Advocate for funding, education, research, and government initiatives aimed specifically at COVID-19-related barriers to care for minorities such as access to testing.[5]

Many argue that the reason for the staggering statistics among America's ethnic minorities is due to higher rates of comorbidities that are known to put those who contract COVID-19 at a higher risk of mortality, hospitalization, and complications from COVID-19. Some argue that it is due to their access to care, lack of insurance, or lack of access to testing. Some argue that it is due to their rate of low socioeconomic status and higher rates of minorities working in essential jobs that do not allow them to stay at home and thus put them at a higher risk for contracting COVID-19. We can see that the reasons for this health care disparity are multifactorial, are complex, and will take a multidisciplinary effort to improve.

In an article calling for action against health inequality with COVID-19-related disparities, the potential reasons for this disparity are discussed as well as the multidisciplinary actions that need to occur to help heal this wound.[4] They note that the people of color are likely to suffer more job loss because of the strains of the pandemic on the economy as 16.8% of Black workers and 17.6% of Hispanic workers are employed in jobs most at risk because of the state of the economy. With this effect on employment, this could further affect more people of color losing their insurance; lack of insurance is a deterrent to seek medical care. People of color receive better care when cared for by providers of the same cultural identity; however, for example, 12% of the US population is Black, but 5% of health care providers are Black. To combat this, it is recommended to form partnerships between schools to educate and expose students to health care occupations in their community (citation?), as well as advocating with local political leaders, hospital administrators to aid in providing mentorship, and financial incentives to reduce economic hardship/barriers to get an education. One such example is the National COVID-19 Dislocated Worker Grant, which provides funds that many Americans are using toward education and learning new skills, thus improving the chance of employment.[3]

Owing to numerous factors such as implicit bias by the medical community and prior history of people of color being failed by the medical system, a lot of people of color distrust medical treatment and medical providers.[4] This distrust can impact the community's perception of risk, leading to myths, misconceptions of risk, and less community involvement in safety measures such as wearing a mask or social distancing. To combat this, recommended interventions include[4]

- Better training programs for health care professionals that represent the cultural makeup of the local communities they serve
- Training program at the institutional and individual level that seek to combat racism, implicit bias, and microaggressions
- Polices in place that mandate interactive training for all staff that not only engages professionals but also recognizes the role of social determinants of health
- Clinicians and health care staff nurturing an environment that embraces cultural humility
- Being advocates for research and funding geared toward patients who experience implicit bias and disparity in health care.

An article published in the *American Journal of Public Health*[5] offered strategies that combat barriers to care for those with COVID-19 in minority communities. With increased testing initiatives during the pandemic, access to testing has not been equivalent across races. Drive-in testing and telehealth screenings have not been accessible because of the lack of technology or transportation. The cost of care continues to be a barrier despite Medicaid/Medicaid and the Families First Coronavirus Response Act. A visit to the ER, beyond testing for COVID-19, can still lead to medical bills, deterring those in the community from seeking care. Partnerships among academic institutions and community organizations to fast-track screening sites and resource testing centers in the areas of need are recommended. There should also be a standard approach to counseling, educating patients of racial communities about health risks to contracting COVID-19, and making sure living conditions are discussed with those that do test positive for COVID-19. It also advised that the US has been researched and drafted COVID-19 response and treatments primarily from China and Italy, 2 countries with populations racially unlike the US. We need to take a closer look at COVID-19 treatment and response strategies with our data or with countries that have populations more like that of the US.

COVID-19 Direct Effect on Non–COVID-19-Related Medical Conditions: the New Health Care Disparity

Patient X was diagnosed with Stage IV rectal melanoma in May. She had to wait 2 months for her colonoscopy which would ultimately make her diagnosis. Because of a delay in diagnosis, she suffered a delay in surgical intervention, immunotherapy, and radiation treatment for her aggressive cancer. She would also find herself in an ER and then be admitted to the hospital because of the complications that could have been avoided had her diagnosis been made sooner. How many other patients faced similar experiences? According to a study conducted by the Epic Health Research Network,[6] the number of screening appointments for cervical, breast, and colon cancer was 86 %–94% lower in the early months of the pandemic than in prior years. In an opinion piece[6] in the New York Times from September 2020, Dr Farrugia (president and CEO of the Mayo Clinic) advised that "in the case of cancer alone, our calculations show we can expect a quarter of a million additional preventable deaths annually if normal care does not resume." In the same opinion piece, Suzanne Steinbaum, DO, a preventive cardiologist and volunteer medical expert for the American Heart Association stated: "I'm seeing patients with preexisting heart problems who've gotten worse and had increases in blood pressure or blood sugar during the shelter in place. Even women without heart problems were eating and sleeping poorly, skipping exercise, and under lots of stress—all of which can contribute to heart disease, the leading cause of death in women in the US."

In May of 2020, canceled/postponed elective surgeries, outpatient procedures, and clinic appointments starting in March were recommended by the US surgeon general, the CDC, numerous medical societies, and state orders across the US.[7] An estimated 4 million elective surgeries would be canceled in the US during 12 weeks of disruption because of COVID-19, according to a study published in the *British Journal of Surgery*.[7] As a result, almost all joint replacements and many preventative cardiac procedures were postponed and a quarter of patients with cancer had delays in their cancer treatments. Routine pediatric vaccination declined and global vaccination campaigns halted, leaving more than 80 million children unvaccinated. Elective procedures may be viewed as optional, but most are not. Procedures such as hysterectomies, cancer biopsies, and knee replacements if delayed can have a devastating impact on quality of life and outcomes.[8]

COVID-19 and its Impact on Cardiac Emergencies

A comparative cross-sectional study[9] was conducted at the Rawalpindi Institute of Cardiology, a tertiary cardiac center of Pakistan, which assessed the impact of COVID-19 on management, admissions, and mortality in their emergent cardiac patients. This study compared the number of emergency department (ED) visits, overall death, admission, cases of decompensated heart failure, ST-Elevated Myocardial Infarctions (STEMIs), and other cardiac emergencies during COVID-19 lockdown to the same time period in 2019 (pre-COVID-19). The results were published in an article by Hamid Sharif Khan and colleagues. During 45 days of lockdown due to the pandemic from March to May, the outpatient department was closed and the hospital was only providing emergency services including percutaneous coronary intervention (PCI) for acute STEMI. It was decided, however, that the stable patient with STEMI and those patients with suspected COVID-19 symptoms would be lysed to prevent the risk of COVID-19 transmission. This study showed a dramatic decline in the admission of cardiac ailments at a tertiary hospital, which demonstrates the impact COVID-19 could have on the morbidity and mortality of cardiac patients. The data from this study are listed later in discussion and highlight the breath of complicated cardiac patients that may be in a worse situation and that will likely present to this hospital once the pandemic is over.

- 32.8% decrease in total ED visits
- 86.86% decrease in admission for decompensated heart failure
- 37.84% decrease in STEMI cases
- 45.33% decrease in overall hospital admission

Decreased Hospital Admissions and Emergency Room Visits Due to the Fear of Contracting COVID-19

A CDC report compared ER visits in April of 2020 with 2019 data, numbers of those presenting to the ED with nonspecific chest pain, myocardial infarction (MI) decreased. ER visits for common atypical symptoms of MI also decreased.[9] Analysis of CDC data demonstrated that in New York and New Jersey from March 15 to May 2,

2020, more than 6000 people died of an MI and more than 800 people died of complications from DM than the same time frame in prior years.

Personal observation

Before I would be furloughed from my position in the ED because of financial hardship COVID-19 placed on my hospital, it was eerie walking in and not having a single patient on the tracking board. Normally, I would walk in for my shift and 5 to 6 patients would be waiting for me to clock in. My first thought was what happened to all the patients with stroke, MI, and other life-threatening pathology that normally present to our ED? We know people did not stop having MIs during the pandemic.

In the United Kingdom during the lockdown, the public message was to stay at home, leaving home for only essential needs just as it was in the US. In the UK and the US in March during the time of lockdown, there was much anxiety among the general public especially those with preexisting conditions. In England alone, there were 29% fewer ED attendances. The Office for National Statistics reported the highest death rate in England and Wales since the year 2000. There were 6082 more deaths than the 5-year average, and only 3475 of these deaths were related to COVID-19,[8] raising more alarm that an increased number of deaths were occurring unrelated to COVID-19 because of the strain on the health care system due and public resistance to see medical attention because of concerns for contracting COVID-19.

Toll on Routine Medical Care

The use of telehealth and virtual visits has proven helpful for many people seeking nonurgent medical care. However, high-risk populations such as minorities and the elderly may not have access to them. High literacy in technology, the Internet, and access to technology capable of accessing telemedicine are needed, in which at-risk patients may have difficulty to accessing.[10] The Israeli Center for Disease Control recommends raising awareness using media campaigns calling for the patient to not neglect acute or chronic medical needs or screenings.[10] They also recommend calling patients in your practice or community who are known to be at risk are equally important to promote community health for COVID-19-related practices and non–COVID-19-related medical needs such as screening and medical appointments.[10]

In the spring, at the start of the pandemic, many hospitals asked patients to stay at home, not seek routine care, and not seek ER care with mild symptoms. The health care system is faced with a fine balance to treat not only those with COVID-19 but also those with non–COVID-19-related medical needs.[8] Ensuring that by focusing on treating and preventing COVID-19, we are not worsening morbidity and mortality for those with non–COVID-19-related medical needs. We must equitably care for both COVID-19- and non–COVID-19-related patients. The IQVIA Institute for Human Data Science estimates there are 42 million mammograms performed annually, with a cancer detection rate of 5.1 per 1000 mammograms performed. Thus, this suggests that for each month, screening mammograms are closed, and 17,850 Americans with breast cancer will be undiagnosed. Short-term limitations may be needed as cases of COVID-19 increase; however, medicine does not know yet the evidence-based risk benefit of short-term closings and if this is needed on an individual basis or as a population.[8]

In an online interview,[11] Tom Lindquist, the CEO of Allina Health-Aeta, advises that besides reaching out to media interviews and recording podcasts encouraging at-risk populations to seek care and encourage patients to return to routine care, they are making efforts to make sure at-risk patients feel safe for their visit. They are sending convenience packages to seniors that include thermometers, masks, and hand sanitizer to help them feel safe to visit a clinic if they need or prefer this option over a virtual visit.

DISCUSSION: WHAT CAN WE DO AS HEALTH CARE PROVIDERS
Key Points

- Provide education to our patients on the risk of contracting COVID-19 during unrelated hospital admission versus the benefit of the hospital admission for non–COVID-19-related illness.
- Discuss COVID-19 with our patients with the truthful data and up-to-date CDC guidelines to prevent transmission are crucial such as wearing a mask, social distancing, and avoiding crowds, just as we counsel them on smoking cessation and wearing their seatbelt.
- Advising and educating patients on the risk benefits of having an elective procedure, being admitted to the hospital versus their actual risk of contracting COVID-19.
- Proactively reaching out to patients, encourage medical screening examinations, their need for urgent, emergent, and routine care while reassuring patients' measures we are doing to ensure their safety.
- Telemedicine and virtual visits have increased access; however, we need to have a way to call or reach our elderly patients and those at risk who may not have access to them to raise awareness for the need for routine, acute, and chronic medical needs

Risk of Nosocomial COVID-19 Infection from Unrelated Hospital Admission

At the start of the pandemic, and still currently, there has been a significant decline in hospital admissions for non–COVID-19-related pathology. This is believed to be partly due to patients' anxiety about contracting COVID-19 and anxiety about the risk of mortality associated with contracting COVID-19 during a hospital stay. One thing we as providers can do to encourage patients to agree to admission or seek emergency medical care is educate and counsel patients that their risk for contracting COVID-19 during a non–COVID-19-related admission, although there is still a risk, is relatively low. Patients being admitted to the hospital actually have a greater risk of contracting COVID-19 in the community than as a nosocomial infection. [12]

The risk of contracting COVID-19 during hospital admission and the risk of mortality was evaluated by the COPE-Nosocomial Study,[12] and results were discussed in an article by Carter and colleagues The study's aim was to identify patients who acquire nosocomial COVID-19 (NC) infection during their hospital admission and their risk of mortality compared with those with community-acquired COVID-19 (CCA) infections. In this observational study, they looked at 1564 patients admitted to the hospital for COVID-19. They compared outcomes between those admitted for a non–COVID-19-related reason within 15 days of diagnosis with those that were not recently admitted to the hospital and thus contracted the virus from the community. Of all 1564 cases they looked at, only 12.5% of the patients contracted COVID-19 from their recent hospital stay. NC infection was associated with lower mortality rate than CAC infections. The median survival time in patients with NC infections was 14 days compared with 10 days in patients with CAC infections. There was no difference between 7-day mortality between the 2 groups. However, those with NC infections required longer hospital stay.

SUMMARY

COVID-19 disproportionately affects people of color in terms of hospital admission, severity of illness, and mortality. This is a multifactorial problem with multiple coordinated events that need to align to help improve the lives of those at risk for COVID-19 not just at the level of the health care delivery system but at the city, state, and federal levels. We need to increase our own training in diversity and promote cultural humility for not only ourselves but also the organizations we work for. We know that COVID-19 is affecting those with non–COVID-19-related medical needs and ultimately increasing morbidity and mortality from non–COVID-19-related medical conditions. We as providers can take simple yet big measures in health promotion and wellness to combat disparities in the face of COVID-19. We need to ensure that our patients are educated on the need to seek help when they need it, continue to receive routine care during the pandemic, and educate our patients on the risk of contracting COVID-19 versus the larger risk of suffering morbidity and mortality from their non–COVID-19-related medical illness. We need to increase health promotion and wellness with our minority patients disproportionally at risk should they contract COVID-19. Not only do we have to increase health promotion around COVID-19 but also we have to ensure that they have access to care and testing and recognize things we can do in our community or practice to ensure they have these capabilities.

CLINICS CARE POINTS

- People of color are at a greater risk for hospitalization, complications, and death from COVID-19. We as medical providers need to increase contact with our patients at risk within our practice and community. We need to incorporate health promotion and wellness around COVID-19 in our patients of color. We need to take measures to ensure they have access to care and testing. We need to ensure our patients of color trust us by promoting cultural humility in our practices.

- There is a fine balance between preventing COVID-19 and treating those who contract COVID-19, while still treating those who need medical screening and have non–COVID-19-related medical needs. We need to incorporate health promotion, wellness, and education to our patients on the need to seek care when they truly need it and the risk/benefit of contracting COVID-19 versus the risk of morbidity and mortality for non–COVID-19-related medical needs.

DISCLOSURE

The author has nothing to disclose.

REFERENCES

1. CDC. Covid-19 cases, hospitalization, and death by race/ethnicity 2020. Available at: https://www.cdc.gov/coronavirus/2019-ncov/downloads/covid-data/hospitalization-death-by-race-ethnicity.pdf. Accessed November 1, 2020.
2. Renelus BD, Khoury NC, Chandrasekaran K, et al. Racial disparities in COVID-19 hospitalization and in-hospital mortality at the height of the New York City pandemic. J Racial Ethn Health Disparities 2020. https://doi.org/10.1007/s40615-020-00928-y.
3. US Department of Labor. Covid-19 dislocated worker grant. Employment and Training Administration; 2020. Available at: https://www.dol.gov/agencies/eta/dislocated-workers/grants/covid-19. Accessed November 1, 2020.

 4. Johnson-Agbakwu C, Ali NS, Oxford C, et al. Racism, COVID-19, and health inequity in the USA; a call to action. J Racial Ethn Health Disparities 2020. https://doi.org/10.1007/s40615-020-00928-y.
 5. Brown IM, Khan A, Slocum J, et al. COVID-19 disparities and the black community: a health equity-informed rapid response is needed. Am J Public Health 2020;110(9):1350–1.
 6. Graves G. The hidden toll of Covid-10. Health 2020;34(7):92–5. Available at: http://cuw.ezproxy.switchinc.org/login?url=http://search.ebscohost.com/login. aspx?direct=true&AuthType=cookie,ip,cpid&custid=s8470807&db=s3h& AN=144860333&site=ehost-live&scope=site. Accessed November 1, 2020.
 7. Nepogodiev D. Elective surgery cancellations due to the COVID-19 pandemic: global predictive modeling to inform surgical recovery plans. Br J Surg 2020; 107(11):1440–9.
 8. Bruno B, Rose S. Patients left behind: ethical challenges in caring for indirect victims of the Covid-19 pandemic. Hastings Cent Rep 2020;50(4):19–23.
 9. Khan HS, Mohsin M, Saif M, et al. Impact of COVID-19 pandemic associated lockdown on admissions secondary to cardiac ailments in a Tertiary Cardiac Center of Pakistan. Pak Armed Force Med J 2020;70(1):S342–6.
10. Saban M, Schachar T. Social distancing and dangers of access block to health care services during COVID-19 pandemic. Emerg Care J 2020;16(9098):63–6.
11. Greene J. 'COVID has actually amplified the reason for value-based care'[Interview]. Detroit: Crain Communications; 2020.
12. Carter B, Collins JT, Barlow-Pay F, et al. J of Hospital Infection. 2020. Available at: https://www-clinicalkey   com.cuw.ezproxy.switchinc.org/#!/content/playContent/ 1-s2.0-S0195670120303443?returnurl=null&referrer=null. Accessed November 1, 2020.

Printed and bound by CPI Group (UK) Ltd, Croydon, CR0 4YY

03/10/2024

01040408-0002